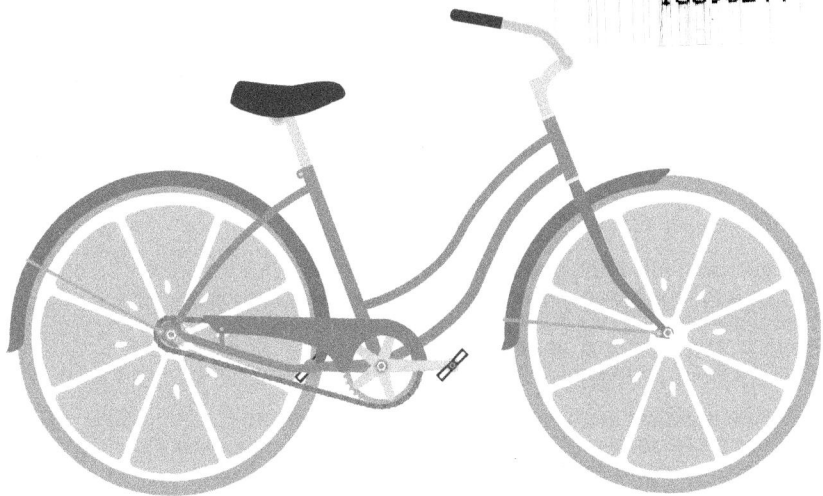

EAT MOVE GROOVE

Unlock the Simple Steps to Lifelong Nutrition, Fitness & Wellness

Susan M. Kundrat

Registered Dietitian Nutritionist

EAT MOVE GROOVE

© 2024 Susan M. Kundrat

This book is written as a source of information only. It is not intended for personal medical advice. The information contained in this book is not a substitute for advice from qualified medical providers. Consult your physician or qualified medical provider before starting any new eating, exercise, or health program. The names of actual clients have been changed to protect privacy.

The trademark for EAT MOVE GROOVE ™ has been applied for.

Library of Congress Control Number: 2024904190

ISBN (paperback): 979-8-9886707-0-4
ISBN (hardcover): 979-8-9886707-1-1
ISBN ebook: 979-8-9886707-2-8
ISBN audiobook: 979-8-9886707-3-5

Editorial services: Sheila Buff; Sandra Wendel, Write On, Inc.

Illustrator: Irina Burtseva

Cover and interior design: Marko Markovic, 5mediadesign.com

Interior design: Kirsten Dennison

Proofreaders: Kristen Roberts; Mary Fleming

Author photo: Holly Birch

Published by Eat Move Groove, PLLC

Website: *www.eatmovegroove.com*

To my mother, Mary Elizabeth Kundrat, English teacher extraordinaire, who inspired me to communicate effectively and challenged me to work hard and reach for my goals—and to all of the amazing teachers who inspire students everywhere to embrace learning and dream big.

Other Books by Susan M. Kundrat

101 Sports Nutrition Tips (2005, 2015)

Training and Conditioning Presents: The Nutrition Edge, a Compilation of the Best Sports Nutrition Articles from Training & Conditioning *Magazine*, editor (2010)

Join our Eat Move Groove community, subscribe to Eat Move Groove, and follow us on your favorite social media channels:

eatmovegroove.com

@eatmovegroove

Eat Move Groove

Eat Move Groove, LLC

Susan Kundrat MS, RDN, LDN

Eatmovegroove2211

Contents

PART I

How to Eat

PART II

How to MOVE

LIST OF RECIPES

Introduction

Here's why this book is different from any other nutrition, fitness, or wellness book you may have read in the past. I've spent my entire career working in the intriguing and ever-growing field of a lifetime: nutrition and well-being. I've worked with people of all ages to help them eat to optimize health, boost energy and fuel activity, and decrease disease risk. In addition to helping consumers of all ages, I've worked with youth athletes, college athletes, Olympic athletes, and professional athletes with sights set on winning an NBA championship. Go Milwaukee Bucks!

I've had countless clients who have learned to eat and move to successfully manage chronic health conditions such as high cholesterol, high blood pressure, and diabetes. I've helped clients eat to get stronger and lose body fat, both to lower their risk of disease and to get them back to enjoying activities they've missed. I've gotten to see how creatively blending eating and moving with a supportive lifestyle can totally change a person's life. I can help you change your life too. It's been an amazing journey, and there's so much more to go.

EAT MOVE GROOVE blends my decades of experience, research, and practical application into a book that can support your well-being on a daily basis.

You'll see that the **2211** (said like this: twenty-two, eleven) EAT plan I offer in this book is a simple plan to implement. It's not a diet. It's a positive way to think about food and enjoy eating. And you'll find that the MOVE plan is just as intuitive. It will help you find ways to move your body that feel good to you and are easy to do. You'll explore all kinds of ideas to support your well-being and boost your health span in the GROOVE part of the book too. With *EAT MOVE GROOVE*, I make it simple, positive, doable, fun, and focused on you.

Thousands of books, programs, websites, podcasts, and plans are focused on diet, exercise, well-being, and weight loss. What makes my EAT MOVE GROOVE plan and **2211** unique? How is this book different from the rest?

This book is for everyone. Maybe, like my client Sharon, you have struggled for what seems like forever to understand how to put the multitude of nutrition and exercise guidelines into practice in your life. Or, perhaps you, like Skye, are on a tight budget and so crunched for time that you don't think there is a way to eat well, move your body, and be able to embrace well-being in your hectic life. You might also understand James, who feels frustrated by not knowing what to eat and how much to exercise to lower his blood pressure, so he throws up his hands in frustration.

I understand the challenges and potential roadblocks that can make embracing a wellness lifestyle difficult. So keep reading. You'll find that this program is much different from any other you may have tried.

EAT MOVE GROOVE is

- Simple
- Flexible
- Positive
- Grounded in science
- Sustainable

How did EAT MOVE GROOVE get its start?

After earning a degree in dietetics while playing basketball at Minnesota State University–Mankato, completing a dietetic internship at Boston's Beth Israel Deaconess Medical Center, and working as a clinical dietitian for two years back in the Midwest, I entered graduate school at Iowa State University to focus on the intersection between human nutrition and physical activity.

I landed a graduate assistantship with a respected nutrition education professor and joined an innovative wellness team on campus to enhance student well-being. I was one of three educators in nutrition, exercise, and psychology who ran the university wellness center for students as part of my training. That's where the idea of EAT MOVE GROOVE began to simmer, more than three decades ago. The combination of nutrition, activity, and the psychology of supporting a wellness lifestyle just clicked for me as a practitioner.

True well-being is holistic. It's not just what we eat and how we move. Well-being encompasses so much more, including building simple habits, developing relationships that support health and wellness, and finding ways that feel good to you to GROOVE every day, whether that's spending time in nature, singing and dancing, or prioritizing a good night's sleep. Our actions are all interconnected.

From my youth, the athlete in me was trained to work cooperatively as part of a team. The clinician in me knew that fostering overall well-being meant so much more than providing nutrition advice. I learned from my academic, clinical, and sports colleagues and was eager to put this holistic view of optimizing well-being into practice.

Later, at the University of Illinois Urbana–Champaign, I started my professional career in sports and wellness nutrition as a member of an enthusiastic, creative team of fitness, nutrition, and injury prevention professionals, where we worked with a crew of students eager to learn from us. The teamwork among us reinforced and boosted my personal philosophy of EAT MOVE GROOVE with the focus on looking at well-being from a panoramic point of view.

Throughout my professional career, I have held many subsequent positions at universities, started and managed a private consulting business with a nutrition, health, and well-being focus, and worked with a wide range of organizations and companies to enhance nutrition and well-being for consumers, athletes, families, corporate teams, and people with a myriad of backgrounds and health concerns.

The secret to a successful positive lifestyle program was always the same: working as a team with experts in nutrition, fitness, and well-being to develop programs and plans that are not only based in solid science, but are practical, positive, and possible to bring to life.

For the past eleven years, I have been fortunate to teach these concepts to students at the University of Wisconsin–Milwaukee with a hands-on learning model. It's so evident that we can learn how to eat and how to move, but without the groove, which includes how we live within our communities every day, optimal well-being isn't complete.

This brings me to writing this book. For years I have wanted to take the basics of nutrition, fitness, and well-being and develop a simple, easy-to-implement, research-based program for consumers of all backgrounds. I have worked with thousands of students, clients, and everyday people who are confused by the conflicting information about how to eat, move, and support their bodies.

EAT MOVE GROOVE is a source for positive, practical, easy-to-practice recommendations based on research from professionals in nutrition, fitness, and well-being. It's a philosophy developed as a lifestyle—not a diet.

This book is a guide for incorporating practical tools into your day to carry out recommendations from decades of research in these areas. And it's simple. Welcome to EAT, MOVE, GROOVE!

Welcome to EAT MOVE GROOVE

Let's get going with the basics. This plan is a positive way to live every day. It's a plan that will help you develop simple daily habits that are easy to implement. When life feels out of control, EAT MOVE GROOVE and the 2211 (twenty-two eleven) plan will be your rock, your stability.

The program is built on solid research in the areas of nutrition, movement, fitness, and well-being. It's flexible, so you can utilize the basics of the plan daily, even when you're extra busy, short on time, traveling, or feeling rundown. When life gets in the way of your well-being (trust me, it does for everyone at times), you can rely on EAT MOVE GROOVE to renew yourself and reconsider your priorities.

I hope you find you can put this plan into practice and enjoy doing it. It's my intention that this book and online support and tips at *eatmovegroove.com* can help you come away with a feeling of "I can do this."

Three Well-Being Foundations

Like anything strong, sturdy, and stable in life, the 2211 lifestyle, the simple plan this book is built around, is resilient. This plan is set up with three well-being foundations: what you EAT, how you MOVE, and how you GROOVE. The GROOVE includes the simple steps you can do to take care of yourself, support your well-being, and also support how you EAT and MOVE. This positive reinforcement and reflection will help you incorporate the 2211 lifestyle into your lifelong norm. By incorporating all three aspects of the plan each day, you'll be gaining the strong, resilient foundation you will rely on to boost longevity.

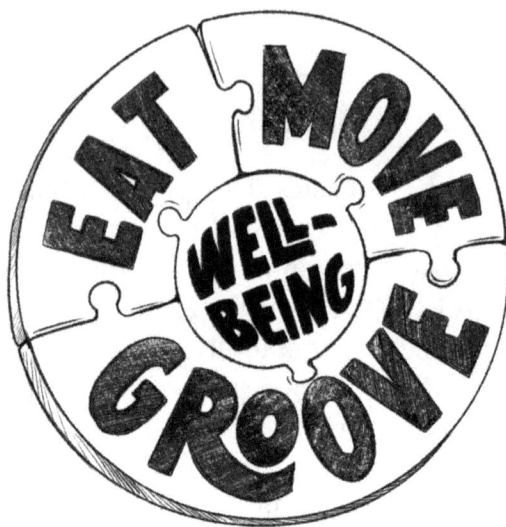

The 2211 Lifestyle

How to Use This Book

You can read this book all at once, or, if you prefer, you can use it as a personal well-being manual, choosing the chapters you are most interested in implementing at any given time.

You'll learn that a little planning—even a few minutes each day—can help you prepare for the day ahead, so it's easy to make decisions to enhance your lifestyle. For example, taking just a few minutes every evening to plan your meals, activity, and time for enjoyment for the next day can make all the difference. That's a gift you can give yourself each day.

It's empowering to know that however you choose to utilize this book, EAT MOVE GROOVE can easily be your lifestyle. And because you don't go on or off this plan, and it just becomes a part of you and supports your well-being, you can add years to your health span (healthy years, not just years).

You might ask yourself: **Why does it sometimes feel so hard to consistently eat well, be active, and manage life?**

The answers we receive can be conflicting, restrictive, and, quite frankly, full of unrealistic recommendations that are difficult to maintain over time. But not EAT MOVE GROOVE. Why?

- EAT MOVE GROOVE is *simple.*
- EAT MOVE GROOVE is *flexible.*
- EAT MOVE GROOVE is *grounded in solid research.*
- EAT MOVE GROOVE is *a lifestyle, not a fad.*
- EAT MOVE GROOVE is *positive.*
- EAT MOVE GROOVE is *sustainable.*

This book is about finding a simple, positive plan you can rely on. It's a plan you can feel confident about and know that it's based on sound practices.

It's organized into five main parts. In chapter 1, you'll learn more about the program, understand how it's set up, and get ready to move ahead.

In Part I, or How to EAT (chapters 2 to 7), you'll learn about the 2211 EAT plan. You'll see how this simple eating plan can be easily incorporated into your days. You'll find tips, recommendations, sample meal plans, and easy-to-make tasty recipes to support your healthy lifestyle, whether you're eating at home or on the go.

In Part II, or How to MOVE (chapters 8 to 10), you'll explore the 2211 MOVE part of the plan and find out how to maintain your well-being and enhance longevity by moving your body in a way that works for you.

In Part III, or How to GROOVE (chapters 11 and 12), you'll understand how to get your groove on, finding ways to support and reinforce your well-being and foster positive behaviors to take care of YOU.

In the References and Resources section, you'll find additional reading to support your EAT MOVE GROOVE plan. Plus, you'll find lots of additional resources online on the book's website at *eatmovegroove.com*.

Now, let's get moving (and grooving) with EAT MOVE GROOVE!

1

The Basics of
EAT MOVE GROOVE

E AT MOVE GROOVE offers you a simple, no-nonsense, practical way to eat, move, and groove every day of your life. Because the program doesn't require you to eat special foods, buy high-end groceries, or eat foods you don't like, you can easily adapt your current eating routine to the plan.

Because *you* choose how you move your body, what feels good to you, and what you like to do, you start with your typical exercise routine and gradually move into or start one with the 2211 MOVE plan. You blend your life *with* the plan—you're not changing your life *for* the plan.

You will find all kinds of ways to get your groove on with this plan. GROOVE brings in positivity, reflection, gratitude, joy, and supportive activities and experiences to help you create a life that is full and meaningful. Choose what works for you. I challenge you to try new activities and join like-minded readers in the EAT MOVE GROOVE online community. Join today at *eatmovegroove.com* and get grooving!

How Do I Eat on the 2211 Plan?

The EAT plan is based on decades of research pointing to a plant-forward eating lifestyle. Plant-forward eating means your meals and snacks are based around plant foods like fruits, vegetables, whole grains, beans and peas, nuts and seeds, and healthy fats like olive oil. A plant-forward eating lifestyle has many well-researched health-enhancing benefits.

Because all foods fit into the 2211 EAT plan, it may include animal foods, such as low-fat dairy, fish, and lean chicken, pork, and beef. You will choose protein-rich foods you enjoy. These might be plant-based proteins like bean burritos. Or you may like a grilled chicken breast, a grilled beef burger, or a yogurt smoothie. No matter what you like to eat, you can still enjoy a plant-forward lifestyle and reap the benefits.

Eating with the 2211 Plan

Every meal starts with 22: 2 cups of produce (fresh, frozen, or canned fruits or vegetables and juices) and at least 2 ounces of protein.

That's 2 servings (2 cups) of fruits or vegetables (either or a mix), plus a 2-ounce (or a bit more) serving of protein.

The 2 cups of vegetables or fruit can be anything you like. To give you an idea, 1 cup of a vegetable is roughly equal to 10 raw baby carrots, 1 medium red bell pepper, 3 stalks of celery, or 10 stalks of asparagus. One cup of fruit is equal to 1 medium apple, pear, or orange, 8 medium strawberries, or about 20 grapes.

Two ounces of protein means 1 cup of cooked black beans, or 2 ounces of low-fat cheese, fish, or lean meat such as turkey, chicken, or roast beef. It's also equivalent to half a cup of nuts or seeds, 2 cups of milk or protein-packed plant-based milks like soy milk or pea protein milk, or 2 eggs.

Then add in the 11, which equals 1 serving of a grain or starch and 1 serving of a healthy fat source.

One serving of a grain or starch might be a slice of whole-grain bread, a cup of unsweetened cereal such as Cheerios, a half cup of cooked rice or pasta, or a small baked potato or sweet potato.

Healthy fats are fats that are good for you, such as a tablespoon of olive oil or half an avocado. Certain foods like plant-based oils, nuts and seeds, and fatty fish like salmon and tuna contain the type of fats that can boost heart health and lower the risk for disease. Choose these fat sources most of the time to boost your overall health and well-being.

2	2 cups of fruits and vegetables
2	2 (or more) ounces of protein
1	1 grain (preferably a whole grain) or starch
1	1 serving of a healthy fat

How Often Do I Eat on the 2211 Plan?

The plan is set up so that you eat three moderate-sized meals a day, plus snacks if you choose. It's important to develop a set eating plan and start your day with a meal to get your body going and fuel yourself with energy at the beginning of the day. By eating the 2211 way, you provide your body with all-important protein to help maintain your lean muscle mass and optimize strength. Eating on a schedule gives you peace of mind that you are optimizing the foods you choose to keep your energy up all day long.

The time of day you eat your meals will vary depending on your daily schedule. For example, you may be a shift worker and eat your "breakfast" at 9:00 p.m. before heading into work. No matter how your days and nights play out, you can plan to eat three meals a day utilizing the 2211 framework and add in snacks too.

Snacks

I'm a big believer in snacks—and there are so many easy options for planning healthy snacks. Learn to listen to yourself and to your personal hunger and fullness cues. If you feel your stomach rumbling, or feel the need for an energy lift, it may be time for a snack. For some people (me included), having a mid-afternoon snack really helps keep energy up during the day. It can also be helpful to plan for a snack after your activity or exercise during the day. This recovery fuel becomes more important when you've been active and when you MOVE.

Eating a balanced snack (a snack with foods containing a mix of protein and carbohydrates) helps your muscles repair tissue and refuel. I like to have some apple slices along with peanut butter on whole wheat crackers. How about a handful of nuts with an orange? Other good choices are a smoothie made with yogurt and frozen fruit or a tortilla with refried beans and salsa. (You can learn more about fast, easy snacks that fit into the 2211 plan at *eatmovegroove.com*.)

Stay hydrated throughout the day by keeping a glass of water or a water bottle close by. Sometimes it's hard to know whether you're hungry or thirsty. So, before you reach for a snack, reach for your water bottle or coffee cup. Getting your fluid level up may make you lose your desire for the snack, or you may end up having a smaller one.

Love Foods

When you have a day when you need a little something extra, top the 2211 EAT plan off with one or two love foods. What are love foods? They're your favorite foods, the ones you love to eat. The key for love foods is to enjoy them, but also be mindful of the amount.

I encourage you to enjoy your love foods in moderation, picking one or two each day. A love food might be an ounce of good dark chocolate. Or perhaps it's a glass of wine with dinner. Maybe you enjoy a scoop of ice cream after lunch or want a few cookies with your snack. Go ahead and have that love food. It's your choice, and you deserve it. Food is to be enjoyed.

Serve Up Your Meal

A super simple way to implement the 2211 EAT plan is to imagine a baseball, a tennis ball, and a golf ball when you think about portions. At each meal, you want to eat 2 baseballs of produce, 1 tennis ball of protein (that's about 2 to 3 ounces), 1 tennis ball of a grain or starch (that's about ½ cup), and a golf ball of healthy fat.

2 baseballs = produce
1 tennis ball = protein
1 tennis ball = grain
1 golf ball = fat

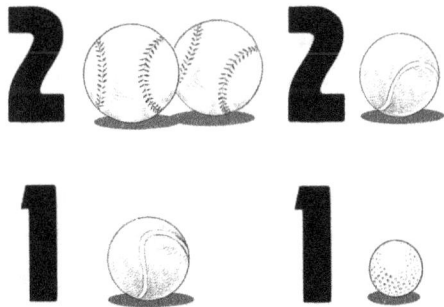

2211 EAT Servings

Customize the EAT Plan

You can easily customize the **2211** EAT plan so it best fits your nutritional needs. For example, your protein needs are based on your body weight and your activity level, so this part of the plan is very flexible. Based on your body's needs, you may opt for more than 2 ounces of protein at a meal. The key is to include a protein source in every meal. (I'll go into that more in the next chapter.)

Put it all together, and a meal could look like this:

✓ 1 orange and 1 cup of broccoli

✓ 3 ounces of chicken breast

✓ 1/2 cup of pasta

✓ 1/2 of an avocado

The Three Macronutrients

Carbohydrate, protein, and fat are macronutrients, sometimes called macros for short. They are the three nutrients in foods that provide energy, or calories.

Carbohydrates are starchy or sugary foods such as fruits, vegetables, bread, pasta, or rice. Carbohydrates are broken down by the body to make blood sugar, also known as glucose, to fuel your body. We need to eat plenty of carbohydrates to provide energy to our bodies. Choosing fruits, vegetables, and whole grains as your primary carbohydrate sources ensures you will be getting important vitamins, minerals, and health-enhancing nutrients every day.

Proteins are your body's building blocks, used to help grow and repair your cells. Protein is found in many plant foods, such as nuts, beans, and tofu and animal foods such as meat, fish, eggs, and dairy products.

Fats from vegetable oils such as olive oil, nuts, seeds, avocados, and some animal foods like eggs are an essential nutrient needed for energy, to promote healthy skin and hair, and to help you absorb vitamins A, D, E, and K. Healthy fats generally come from plants, such as olive oil, avocado oil, or canola oil. While you may enjoy an occasional pat of butter on your baked potato, go for plant-based fats most of the time.

Some foods are mostly protein, carbohydrate, or fat, but most foods are a mix of macronutrients.

High-Carbohydrate Foods

- Fruits and fruit juices
- Vegetables and vegetable juices
- Bread, tortillas, bagels, and cereal bars
- Oatmeal, granola, and other cereals
- Pasta, rice, couscous, and other grains
- Potatoes, sweet potatoes, corn, and peas
- Beans and lentils (also high in protein)
- Milk and yogurt
- Desserts and sweets

High-Protein Foods

- ✔ Beans and lentils
- ✔ Soy foods such as edamame and tofu
- ✔ Nuts, seeds, and nut butters
- ✔ Eggs
- ✔ Milk, yogurt, and cheese
- ✔ Plant-based milks
- ✔ Beef, pork, and lamb
- ✔ Chicken and turkey
- ✔ Fish

Healthy Fats

- ✔ Olive oil
- ✔ Canola, sunflower, safflower, and grapeseed oil
- ✔ Avocado oil
- ✔ Avocados
- ✔ Nuts and nut butters
- ✔ Nut oils such as walnut, peanut, or macadamia oil
- ✔ Seeds such as sunflower seeds, chia seeds, and flax seeds

Can I Really Eat Any Foods with the 2211 Plan?

YES! You can eat any *and* all foods you like to eat on this plan. No kidding. When a food plan is too restrictive, it's our nature to overeat the foods that are forbidden. Plus, let's be honest. We all have our personal likes and dislikes when it comes to food. We also like to eat a variety of different foods. Optimal eating is about so much more than just nutrition. It's also about eating foods we like, eating foods that mean something to us, eating foods that are culturally significant to us, eating foods that elicit fond memories, and eating foods that make us feel good.

So, with the 2211 plan, you have no restriction on the specific foods you eat. As you'll see with the plan, when you eat the 2211 way, you'll be satisfied and won't feel deprived of your favorite foods. By listening to what you want to eat, and being mindful of balanced eating, you can more easily pay attention to your body and respond to it in a positive way.

Are You Serious?

Yes, I am. You can include any foods you want. With the 2211 plan, you eat in moderation, not with restrictions. Food is meant to be enjoyed. The 2211 lifestyle offers the balance between eating in moderation and eating foods you genuinely love to eat.

Let me clarify something. We eat real food, not just calories, grams, macros, or nutrients. While the 2211 EAT plan is highly nutritious, it's also very flexible. This plan is meant to be yours for your life, not just for a few weeks or months. That means everything you learn will provide the basis for your ongoing life of well-being. And well-being includes all your favorite foods.

Will I Lose Weight?

You may lose weight. However, weight loss isn't the primary focus of EAT MOVE GROOVE. If weight loss is one of your reasons for utilizing the 2211 plan, you may well lose weight as a result of implementing the plan. For many people, eating more fruits and vegetables, opting for protein at every meal, and being aware of food portions can foster weight loss. Depending on your starting weight and how your body adapts to this new way of eating, you may find you lose weight.

For many people, the EAT plan is lower in calories than their previous eating pattern, which may result in weight loss. The truth is that we all respond differently to changes in how we eat. Plus, so many factors go into weight loss that it's difficult to predict how dietary changes will affect you. We know from research in this area that some people lose weight more quickly than others, even when they eat the same food plan and get the same amount of exercise. There are many variations in how our bodies adapt to a change in how we eat and our activity level.

That's why on the 2211 plan, we focus on developing sound, easy-to-maintain eating habits.

By doing this, even if your weight changes (or doesn't change), you have developed a plan to maximize your health. That's more important than how much you weigh.

Based on the principles of the 2211 plan, we know that the EAT MOVE GROOVE plan can:

- Lower your risk for disease
- Help you get stronger and maintain physical function and fitness
- Provide your body with an opportunity to boost health, enhance well-being, and foster a positive mindset
- Lower your stress around food and moving your body so you can enjoy eating and feel good moving

Set Healthy Weight-Loss Expectations

If losing weight is one of your goals, healthy weight loss for most people is losing no more than 1 to 2 pounds per week. This is based on scientific research that looks at sensible, reasonable weight loss. That's weight you can lose but also keep off for the long term.

Many factors play into weight loss, including stress, hormones, your personal genetics, your weight loss and gain history, how much muscle you have, your hydration status, medications you take, and simply how your body adapts to different foods and activities.

When you're following a healthy weight-loss eating plan, it's typical to lose weight one week, and maybe not the next. Some people may lose weight faster or slower, but, on average, if the plan lowers your calories, boosts your activity—or both—weight loss will be gradual.

As you get stronger, feel better, and become more accustomed to the plan, you may want to increase your activity, which can enhance body fat loss. If losing 1 to 2 pounds per week sounds slow, that's OK. Slower is better when it comes to weight loss. It gives your body a chance to adapt to weight changes.

If you lose weight at a slower, more consistent pace while also being active and eating in a way to support your muscles, you will lose more body fat and maintain more of your muscle mass and bone. That's our goal with 2211: gradual, healthy changes in your body that improve your health and well-being for the short term and long term. Those gradual changes may also include weight loss.

It's critical to be able to sustain a lifestyle that fosters your well-being. EAT MOVE GROOVE is a lifestyle you can adopt for good. That's another reason the plan is focused on building a positive, balanced lifestyle instead of on weight loss.

Getting Healthier, Not Necessarily Thinner

Not everyone wants to or needs to lose weight. For many people, the goal isn't weight loss but adopting and maintaining a healthy lifestyle. That's why the focus of this program is optimizing health and well-being. Weight loss may be a part of that, but it's not the primary focus of the 2211 plan.

In my experience with clients who adopt the 2211 lifestyle, some do so in part to lose weight or to fit better in their clothes (lose inches). Most importantly, they adopt the plan to have more energy, feel stronger, feel more confident and positive about their health, do the things they want to do each day, and feel empowered to support their personal well-being. There's no question that embracing this lifestyle plan has an abundance of benefits well beyond any number on a scale.

And remember: Your weight alone may have little to do with your overall health and well-being. That's based much more on your lifestyle: what you EAT, how you MOVE, and how you GROOVE day after day.

What about the MOVE Plan?

When I talk about maximizing overall health and well-being, it's all about feeling energized and strong. You don't have to be a world-class body builder. You don't even have to lift heavy weights. But for our bodies to function at their best, we need to put time and attention into moving them, so we breathe a little more heavily (22 or more minutes a day) and also build strength, stability, and flexibility (11 or more minutes a day). It includes getting up and moving during the day to boost your overall movement.

Moving to maintain cardiorespiratory fitness and strength throughout life has many positive benefits. It helps us enjoy moving our bodies all day long, whether that's walking around a park, picking up kids, or enjoying a sunset bike ride. It gives us stability and enhances our balance. It gives us confidence as we move through our day. It helps our bodies burn more calories every day. It helps us age well and avoid frailty.

And moving makes you feel good. Regardless of your age, eating and moving to support your body helps you keep better balance, stay more independent, and enjoy life activities. Eating and moving to foster strong, capable muscles and bones keeps the cells of our bodies going. That's why EAT MOVE GROOVE will guide you to eat well, stay well, and nurture yourself.

Moving your body as much as you can within your personal abilities and opportunities is essential for overall good health and well-being no matter what stage of life you are in. You may have limitations that make some types of activities or exercise impossible or more difficult than others. That's OK. With EAT MOVE GROOVE you'll learn to move your body in ways you can consistently manage and enjoy. You'll explore many different ideas and options for you, but the bottom line is to get moving. With the **2211** lifestyle, the activity piece is your choice too.

Move 33 Minutes (22 + 11) a Day or More

The MOVE plan includes moving three ways during the day:

- MOVE at least **22** minutes a day in a way that boosts your heart rate and gets you breathing more heavily (aerobic activity) per day. That's equal to at least 154 minutes per week.
- MOVE at least **11** minutes a day doing strength/ stretching/stability activities. That's equal to at least 77 minutes per week.
- MOVE often during the day, getting up at least once an hour to walk, stretch, or take a movement break.

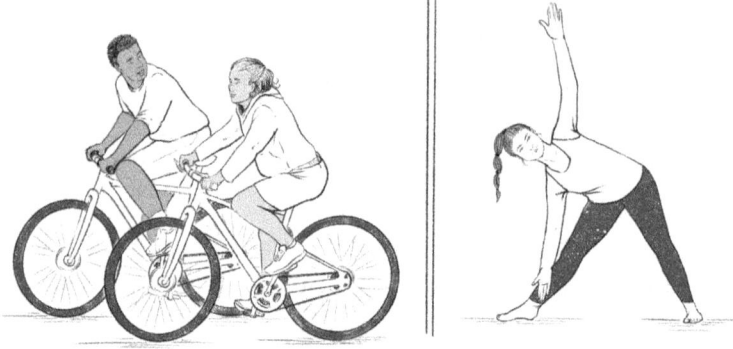

The 2211 MOVE Plan

With the MOVE plan, you'll move your body using your cardiorespiratory system (making your heart beat harder and breathing heavier) for at least 22 minutes a day. If you're new to exercising, start with small bouts of exercise, three or four minutes at a time, to get used to moving more. Gradually work up to 22 minutes of activity a day on most days of the week. You'll find many simple MOVE recommendations, plans, videos, and tips at *eatmovegroove.com*.

If you're already exercising a few days a week, aim to add more activity days. The goal is to get at least 22 minutes a day of feeling your heartbeat higher than usual over most days.

Strengthen 11 Minutes a Day

Here's where the 11 in **2211** MOVE comes into play. In addition to your 22 minutes of daily activity that pumps your blood and boosts cardiovascular health, add in 11 minutes of strength, stability, and stretching exercises that build your muscles and improve your ability to do your normal daily activities.

Move Throughout the Day

As you'll see, moving throughout the day (ideally, every hour for a break from sitting) provides additional health benefits.

Because moving your body each day provides more benefits than just burning calories, with the 2211 lifestyle, you'll be employing the 2211 MOVE plan every day. It will become your norm. You'll enjoy being more active, and you'll notice the benefits of being stronger when you do things like carry in groceries, work in the garden, or walk up the stairs.

You get the most benefit from being more active if you do it most days a week. You'll sometimes have a day when you just don't feel like moving. That's OK. A day to chill and rest now and then won't matter, as long as you're consistent over the long term. If you aren't active currently, don't worry. If you're active some days but not others, that's OK too. You can gradually add activity to your day. Start small—a few minutes a day a few times a day is an ideal beginning.

On the 2211 MOVE plan, you'll find activities that feel good to you, bring you joy, and relieve stress. The activities you enjoy will be different from someone else, so it's important to listen to yourself and incorporate movements that feel good to you. Later in this book, we'll explore fun activities that are easy to do.

Simple Exercises

You have so many ways to boost your well-being with 2211 MOVE options. One terrific way is to use exercise breaks when you have natural shifts in your day. For example, you might get up for a break from working at your desk, or you might have time to recalibrate your morning after the kids start school. Remember that even short periods of activity throughout the day can give you a lift and count toward your daily movement goal. Exercise breaks don't take a lot of time. You can easily fit them into the natural breaks in your day.

In later chapters, I'll teach you how to take a quick break when watching your favorite TV show. I'll also show you some simple ways to practice strength training at your desk. You'll learn how to practice balance exercises next to a table. You can even do a few strength exercises when you brush your teeth or dry your hair. And how about taking a movement break when the soup is warming up on the stove? The opportunities are endless.

As you build your **2211** activity plan into your lifestyle, you may find you have the time to add activity boosts to your **2211** plan. You could plan a 33-minute biking break or even a 44-minute swim on some days. The most important point is to consistently stay active by moving at least 22 minutes per day where you are breathing heavier than normal and at least 11 minutes a day to boost your strength, stability, and flexibility.

What's the Best Movement for Me?

The answer to that question depends on what activities you enjoy and what you find you can incorporate into your lifestyle on a daily basis and keep doing as the years go by.

Ask yourself: What activities make me feel alive and full of energy? Which activities and exercises boost my mood? What do I do that makes me feel strong? In what ways can I move that help me feel more flexible? What makes me feel more powerful? These activities may change over time or even from week to week.

There are so many ways to enjoy an activity in a day, even if you don't consider it "exercise." You might play at the park with your kids or grandkids, walk with a friend to catch up on each other's lives, or garden. Perhaps you would have fun joining a free exercise class online or dancing to music from your favorite artist. Even grocery shopping can be a fantastic way to move if you keep a good pace at the store.

Meet a friend, family member, colleague, or fitness expert to be active with. As you'll see in the third leg of 2211, finding support and reinforcing your positive changes are essential to success. When we feel less stressed and more empowered, we're much more apt to carry that over to our eating and activities.

Get in the GROOVE

GROOVE, the third leg of this well-being plan, is every bit as important as EAT and MOVE. Eating well and moving are cornerstones of science-based, well-being programs. But it's also critical to feel good about what you're doing. There are so many ways to foster your personal health and well-being and fuel your health span besides how you eat and exercise. Because the EAT MOVE GROOVE plan is a lifelong lifestyle, finding ways you GROOVE not only will support how you EAT and MOVE, but grooving is essential to taking care of you. You'll learn many helpful ways to get into your personal GROOVE.

Think of GROOVE as the positivity part of the plan. You'll learn about ways to support yourself and find simple tips for adding more GROOVE to your days. This may mean practicing a few minutes of mindfulness. It might be taking a minute or two out of your day to slow down and breathe deeply. Maybe it's relaxing by reading an enjoyable book. Or perhaps it's catching up with an old friend over coffee. It might be taking a calming bath, listening to your favorite music, enjoying a few moments of quiet, watching a sunset, or setting aside time to focus on your spiritual well-being.

What's important is that you do something just for you every day. When we feel good about ourselves and take care of ourselves, we build the framework to support our personal well-being venture.

Taking time when you can during your day to relax and enjoy life is of utmost importance with the 2211 lifestyle. You may find it's helpful to insert options for reflection into your day. That may equate to giving yourself time to reflect on your day and on the good things that are happening. Some people gain much from a short meditation. Perhaps you start your day with a few moments of contemplation or quiet time. Or maybe you keep a gratitude journal, where you reflect on and write down what you are grateful for at the end of each day.

Your personal positivity practices are up to you and should enhance your experience with 2211. I encourage you to try many different options for this leg of 2211. By taking the time to connect with yourself and others in a positive way, you're reinforcing your worth each day. You're making consistent changes to enhance your health and well-being. You deserve to take a few moments each day to calmly reflect and re-energize.

Finding ways every day to take care of you is at the core of this program. As you read on, you'll find many positive options for support with the 2211 plan.

What If I'm on a Budget?

Because you choose the foods you eat with 2211, you choose where and how to set up your meals. You can certainly eat utilizing the 2211 lifestyle in restaurants, but you can also eat based on the 2211 lifestyle by shopping at bargain grocery stores. When you put your own meals together with your own food, you tend to save a lot of money. You can season food with less salt and more herbs and spices too.

If you like to cook, that's also encouraged. The 2211 lifestyle nutrition plan is so flexible that you can easily implement it on a tight budget with inexpensive, simple-to-make meals and snacks. If you don't like to cook, you'll still find the 2211 plan is easy to implement on a budget. In chapter 5 I'll teach you how to put meals together using packaged and prepared foods instead of cooking from scratch. It's a fast, easy, and relatively inexpensive way to eat well with less cooking.

Eating well and being active doesn't mean spending a lot of money. This program will teach you cost-saving tips to help you manage your food budget while embracing the health benefits of 2211. The option of wellness on a budget makes the 2211 lifestyle accessible to everyone. Everyone deserves to eat well, move their body in ways they enjoy, and enhance their well-being. Cost shouldn't be a barrier for accessing optimal well-being.

In this book and on the *eatmovegroove.com* website, you'll also find many ways to MOVE on a budget. You'll find simple, easy options for moving at home, at work, inside, outside, and on the run. You'll also learn about free and inexpensive online videos and classes with many movement ideas.

There are so many ways to GROOVE that don't cost a penny. While supporting your personal health and well-being is priceless, finding your GROOVE is free and available to you any time.

Meeting Your Health Goals

The 2211 lifestyle is set up to be flexible and easy to implement. It can easily be modified or fine-tuned to meet most health goals. It's also a valuable tool for improving your management of many medical concerns, such as high cholesterol, type 2 diabetes, or high blood pressure.

The plan is set up to facilitate improvements in overall well-being and to decrease your risk of developing common health concerns, such as heart disease, which may be related to diet, exercise, and stress.

Many diseases are related to inflammation in the body. By adopting the 2211 lifestyle, you're eating at least six cups of fruits and vegetables a day. Eating more produce is one of the simplest ways to boost key nutrients, add fiber, and keep calories low. Fruits and vegetables are also high in antioxidants and polyphenols, which are food components that can help lower inflammation and reduce your risk of disease.

You may have already modified your diet or activity program to accommodate specific needs related to medical concerns like arthritis, osteoporosis, high cholesterol, high blood pressure, reflux disease, Parkinson's disease, or celiac disease. You can continue and even improve on those dietary and activity modifications on the 2211 lifestyle. That's where the flexibility of the plan really shines.

Think of the 2211 lifestyle as an added support system for you as you navigate your specific health concerns. You'll read more about working with your healthcare team and using the 2211 plan to meet your personal health and well-being goals in chapter 4.

With the 2211 lifestyle, you'll be supported with free sample meal plans, recipes, grocery lists, and nutrition tips. You'll find articles and videos online on our website, *eatmovegroove.com*. You'll also find recommended online resources that will help you achieve your activity goals. And we'll draw on well-respected experts in the fields of nutrition, exercise, positivity, stress management, mindfulness, and health and wellness coaching for suggestions to help you achieve your goals.

Finding Your Why

What is your *why* for picking up this book? What fuels your personal interest in nutrition, activity, and well-being? Is it to feel better and have more energy? Is it to maintain your overall health? Is it to lower your risk of disease, or manage a medical concern? Is it to get stronger or improve your balance? Is it to lose weight?

Many books have been written on finding your why. Kent Burns describes finding your why as a treasure hunt in his book *What's Your Why?* I like to think of finding your why as an opportunity to stop, look, and listen to yourself. What resonates with you? What purpose do you have for supporting your health and well-being? Why is that important to you personally? I'm convinced that the simple 2211 lifestyle plan with EAT MOVE GROOVE can help you answer that question and provide the tools and support to move forward in a positive way.

To start exploring your why, consider the following checklist. Which of these whys resonate with you?

What's Your Why?

I want to—

- ☐ Feel better
- ☐ Have more energy
- ☐ Eat better
- ☐ Be more active
- ☐ Get stronger
- ☐ Move more easily and confidently
- ☐ Lose weight
- ☐ Feel less stressed
- ☐ Have structure
- ☐ Have a plan
- ☐ Have support
- ☐ Be more balanced
- ☐ Lower my cholesterol
- ☐ Lower my blood pressure
- ☐ Manage my arthritis
- ☐ Manage another medical condition
- ☐ Eat a plant-forward diet in part to care for the environment
- ☐ Find a simple way to reset when life gets out of control

Understanding your whys will help you so much as you develop your personal well-being lifestyle. When we keep our whys top of mind, we EAT, MOVE, and GROOVE to support ourselves every day.

Once you ponder your whys, consider that EAT MOVE GROOVE offers you the how to match your why. What I mean by this is that once you determine your why, you can rely on EAT MOVE GROOVE, our experts, and our support to help you with the how during each and every day. This book and the supporting online program give you the how so you can take the next step toward making simple, lasting, health-enhancing lifestyle changes.

Revisit your whys often to remind yourself of why you're committed to boosting your personal well-being in a positive way. Remind yourself that you have good reasons for finding simple ways to maximize your eating, moving, and grooving. These reminders help us stay focused on why even when life feels out of control, upside down, or full of stress. The why will still be there, even when it's sometimes covered up by life itself.

Finding Your How

Knowing your hows for building and maintaining this lifestyle is just as important as understanding your whys.

In fact, your hows determine your GROOVE. For example, you may enjoy cooking a meal as a way to de-stress after a long day. So, for you, a how is being creative with food in the kitchen. Or perhaps adding a premade salad to a frozen meal is your preference. Cooking might not be your how, but maybe playing table tennis with your kids is more like it.

Your how may be different from other people's hows, and that's good.

What's Your How?

I like to—

- ☐ Grocery shop weekly
- ☐ Pick up groceries when I need them
- ☐ Have groceries delivered to me
- ☐ Cook my own meals
- ☐ Eat out at restaurants
- ☐ Get food at a drive-through
- ☐ Order take-out food
- ☐ Order prepackaged meals or meal kits delivered to me
- ☐ Eat at home
- ☐ Eat on the run
- ☐ Eat fresh cooked meals
- ☐ Eat packaged meals and add to them
- ☐ Eat three meals a day
- ☐ Snack throughout the day
- ☐ Eat with friends or family
- ☐ Eat alone

- ☐ Exercise at home
- ☐ Exercise at a gym
- ☐ Exercise outside
- ☐ Exercise inside
- ☐ Do short bursts of activity several times a day
- ☐ Do longer exercise bouts once a day
- ☐ Exercise watching television
- ☐ Exercise with others
- ☐ Exercise on my own
- ☐ Exercise to music
- ☐ Exercise when it's quiet
- ☐ Meditate
- ☐ Be in nature
- ☐ Enjoy time with my favorite people
- ☐ Walk my dog
- ☐ Breathe deeply
- ☐ Listen to music
- ☐ Laugh

Putting It All Together

The essential elements of EAT MOVE GROOVE are easy to follow.

The **2211 EAT** plan includes the following with each meal:

- 2 cups of fruits or vegetables
- 2+ ounces of protein
- 1 grain portion (whole grains best) or starch
- 1 healthy fat portion

The daily **2211 MOVE** plan includes:

- 22 minutes of movement (aerobic activity) and
- 11 minutes of strengthening, stability, and stretching movement.
- Taking movement breaks every hour.

The **2211 GROOVE** plan is daily support for your personal well-being and includes anything that brings you joy and enhances your health inside and out. That might include:

- Taking a gratitude break
- Volunteering in your community
- Giving yourself positive feedback

To sum it all up, here's why **EAT MOVE GROOVE** is for you:

- It's simple.
- It's easy to implement.
- It's positive.
- It works!

PART I

How to Eat

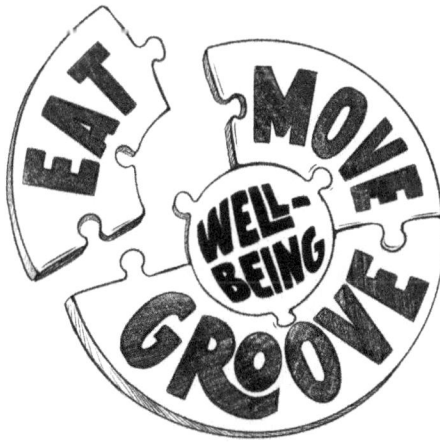

2

How to Eat:
The 2211 Food Framework

The 2211 EAT plan is a straightforward way to plan your meals and eat in a balanced, low-stress, easy way.

Here's what **2211** means to you on this plan. For each meal, you eat 2 cups of fruit or vegetables (or a combination), at least 2 ounces of protein, 1 grain or starch serving, and 1 healthy fat.

The **2211** EAT plan is a plant-forward eating design. Most of what you eat will be plant-based foods simply because meals will contain your choice of fruits, vegetables, grains, and healthy fats. That's good for your health and good for the environment at the same time.

In addition, I encourage eating one or two daily love foods—delicious foods you really enjoy. After all, food is to be savored. You may enjoy a cookie after lunch or a beer with your burger. Your love foods are built into the plan.

The 2211 plan isn't a calorie-counting program. While some foods do have more calories, or energy, than other foods in the same food group, you don't have to choose the lower-calorie options. Of course, if weight loss is on your why list, you may decide to go for fewer calories, but it's entirely up to you. The plan will still work for you. Similarly, if you want higher-energy foods because you're feeling hungry, or if you're getting stronger and gaining muscle mass, you can choose larger portions of all foods.

There will be days when you eat less, and days when you eat more. There will be days when you hit your serving targets with the 2211 plan, but other days may be more challenging. The beauty of the 2211 plan is that it provides a consistent and flexible structure. Use the plan as a guide most of the time, and you'll see the benefits even if you have some days when it's just not possible to follow the plan.

Our overall health and well-being are determined by what we eat, how we move, and how we support ourselves most of the time. We all have days that are extra hectic, days we might not have certain foods available, or days when being active isn't on the schedule.

Our bodies respond to what we do on a weekly and monthly basis, not to what we do only on one or a few days. When we build a foundation that is pointed toward optimizing our well-being most of the time, we're in a good place.

In other words, you may have a rough day or two here or there—or maybe a challenging few weeks—but you can always come back to the 2211 plan. The remarkable thing about the 2211 plan is that it provides opportunities to build on your well-being foundation at every meal and every day. You don't need to stew about yesterday or the week before or the month before. You have today.

Why Love Foods?

One reason I became a Registered Dietitian is because I love food. I love to eat diverse kinds of foods, I love to cook different foods, I love to learn about food and culture, I love to help others eat well and enjoy it, and I love to eat a wide variety of foods. That's why I enthusiastically encourage eating foods you love to eat every day with the 2211 plan. If you love foods that are considered treats, I encourage you to choose one or two to eat every day. Because you'll be eating a very high-quality diet every day with the 2211 plan, you have room to add a treat or two such as dessert, your favorite beverages, or your favorite snack foods.

Besides . . .

- Food is meant to be enjoyed.
- Food is meant to be appreciated.
- Food is meant to be explored.
- Food is our friend, not our enemy.

On the 2211 plan, I suggest adding one or two love foods a day. Listen to your desires for specific foods. Do you want something sweet? How about something salty? Would you enjoy a cocktail with dinner? I think of love foods as foods we are mindful of, and eat in moderation, but also enjoy. Being intuitive about your eating—making peace with your eating and eating all foods—is a critical piece of the 2211 plan.

You can enjoy your love foods but still be mindful of portions. For example, a handful of potato chips might be just what you need with lunch, but being mindful to put the bag away after one serving is also important. When you know you can enjoy love foods, you know that no foods are off limits with the 2211 plan. You know that your love foods are extras to be enjoyed in moderate portions, but this also keeps you from feeling deprived.

Sometimes it's difficult to know how much is enough when you're eating a love food. And sometimes, once we get started, it's hard to stop. Think of a love food as a bonus food when you have a taste for something specific. If one of your reasons for adopting a new eating plan is to maintain or lose weight, I suggest keeping your love food portion to around 100 calories if that feels like enough to you. Check the food labels on your favorite treats so you know how many calories are in one serving. Enjoy your love foods and give yourself a moment to appreciate it. That can help with feeling satisfied with smaller portions.

Your Daily Food Intake

All 2211 meals (including breakfast) contain the following:

2	cups of fruits and vegetables
2	(or more) ounces of protein
1	grain serving (preferably a whole grain) or starch
1	serving of a healthy fat

Here's an example of a simple daily food intake for three meals.

Breakfast

- 2 scrambled eggs with 1 cup sautéed spinach and green onions (2 ounces protein and 1 produce serving)
- 1 cup sliced strawberries (1 produce serving)
- 1 slice whole-grain toast with 1/2 of an avocado (1 grain serving + 1 fat serving)
- Coffee or tea

Lunch

- 1/2 whole-wheat pita with 1/2 cup hummus, 1 slice Provolone cheese, and sliced tomatoes (1 grain serving + 2 ounces protein + 1 produce serving + 1 healthy fat)
- 1 cup canned pears (1 produce serving)
- Iced tea

Dinner

- 2 to 4 ounces grilled salmon (2 to 4 ounces protein + 1 healthy fat)
- 2 cups steamed broccoli and carrots (2 produce servings)
- 1/2 cup roasted potatoes (1 grain/starch serving)
- 5 ounces red wine (1 love food)

Adding Snacks

Snacks are welcome with the 2211 plan. Adding a snack during the afternoon can be especially helpful if you find yourself ravenous by dinner time. If you get hungry between meals, start your snack with produce and protein. That way, you boost your nutrients even more with every snack. Adding protein to fruits and veggies helps you feel full and satisfied. (Check out the snack ideas in chapter 7 and on *eatmovegroove.com*.)

Eating foods high in protein (such as nuts, beans, yogurt, meat, or fish) helps satisfy your hunger—you feel satiated with a relatively small portion. When you add a fruit or vegetable to the protein food, your snack is even more filling, plus you're getting the nutritional benefit of an extra produce portion. You also get the added benefit of additional fiber. Fiber (the nondigestible parts of foods like fruits, vegetables, and grains) also makes us feel more full when we eat.

Snacks can be anything you like but consider adding snacks that contain both produce and protein for the biggest benefit. For example—

- 1 orange with a slice of whole-grain toast and peanut butter
- 1 cup of canned peaches with a handful of almonds
- 1 cup of strawberries with 1/2 cup of Greek yogurt
- 1 cup of baby carrots with 1/2 cup of hummus
- 1 apple with a mozzarella cheese stick
- Smoothie with 1 cup of frozen fruit, 1/2 cup of soy yogurt, and 1/2 cup of 100 percent fruit juice

Fiber

Fiber is the nondigestible part of foods and is found in fruits, vegetables, beans and peas, and grains. You might think of it as the roughage you eat that passes through you. Eating the 2211 way also means eating a high-fiber diet. Choosing a wide range of fruits, vegetables, and whole grains adds fiber to every meal. Plant-based foods high in protein such as beans, soy foods like edamame and tempeh, and nuts and seeds are also great sources of fiber. Most Americans eat about half of the fiber they need in a day, but the 2211 plan is high in fiber.

When you eat more fiber, you help yourself in so many ways. Here are just a few:

- Adding more fiber or bulk to your meals helps you feel full faster and stay full longer. This keeps you satisfied and supports weight management.

- Eating a high-fiber diet can keep your digestive tract working well, as you move food along faster, which is good for your gut and good for you. Insoluble fiber found in whole wheat, leafy greens, seeds, and brown rice can keep your digestive system moving along.
- The bacteria in our digestive system (the microbiome) are fed with a high-fiber diet. Foods high in prebiotic fiber such as bananas, leeks, onions, and berries are great options.
- Eating more fiber can help manage blood sugar levels and blood cholesterol levels. Soluble or gummy fibers found in oatmeal, apples, nuts, and beans are especially helpful.
- Eating a high-fiber diet is associated with a lower risk of having heart disease and certain cancers.

What to Drink

Start your day by drinking at least 22 ounces of fluid (that's almost 3 cups) in the first two hours after waking, no matter the time of day. When we sleep, we get dehydrated, so it's important to rehydrate early in the day. On the 2211 plan, fluids include anything except alcohol or sugary beverages. Water, coffee, tea, 100 percent fruit juice, vegetable juice, milk, almond milk, oat milk, smoothies, or any other fluids you enjoy are included.

The sooner you rehydrate in the morning, the better you will function during the day. Think of your morning rehydration as your morning reset.

Our bodies also function better overall if we are hydrated. After you hydrate early in the day, stay hydrated all day long. Staying hydrated enhances digestion and absorption. That means your body can digest food better, and you benefit from getting the nutrients from food into your cells to boost health and well-being.

Next, drink fluids on a schedule. Our bodies are hydrated when we drink enough to go to the bathroom every few hours and have ample urine that is clear or light-colored. At a minimum, drink half a fluid ounce of water or other liquids daily for every pound you weigh. If you weigh 200 pounds, for example, that's a minimum of 100 ounces of fluid, or about 3 quarts or 12 8-ounce cups. If you weigh 150 pounds, that's a minimum of 75 ounces of fluid a day, or about 2.3 quarts or 9 8-ounce cups.

The easiest way to track your fluid intake and stay hydrated through the day is to fill up 3 24-ounce water bottles or tall glasses. Drink one in the morning and then two throughout the day and into the evening to make sure you're getting your baseline fluid and add other fluid options you enjoy.

Fluids with calories, like most coffee drinks, juices, milk, smoothies, shakes, or any alcoholic drinks, are included in your **2211** meal servings. Water, black coffee, tea, herbal tea, and calorie-free beverages like sparkling water or sugar-free sodas provide fluids, but not calories or energy, so they don't count as **2211** food servings.

If losing weight or maintaining weight are in your why, I suggest keeping fluids high in sugars or with added sugars to a minimum. These drinks (examples are juice drinks, lemonade, fruit punch, sweetened drinks, sodas, and flavored coffee drinks) add extra calories.

For a simple nutrition boost, drink tea. You can maximize your health while also staying hydrated. Drink 2 to 3 cups a day of unsweetened brewed green or black tea to boost your heart health. Special compounds called flavonoids in these teas provide health-enhancing benefits including supporting heart health.

Enjoy herbal teas too. Some teas offer specific benefits as well. Chamomile tea may help you relax and improve sleep. Peppermint tea may help ease an upset stomach. If you prefer iced tea, that's fine too. Once you brew the tea, chill it, or pour it over ice and enjoy.

Now that you have the base of the **2211** EAT plan set up, it's time to dig more deeply into how to use the **2211** EAT plan to put meals together—no matter where you are. In the next chapter, you'll start to make your plan come to life. You'll find that the focus on simple and practical comes into play right away.

3

The 2211 Food Plan

Now that you know what the 2211 EAT plan is, it's time to understand how to combine foods each day using the simple 2211 plan. With the 2211 plan, you'll eat in a plant-forward way. You still eat all the foods you enjoy, including meat and dairy if you prefer, but emphasize eating mostly plant-based foods like fruits, vegetables, grains, beans, nuts, and seeds. Start with your favorite foods in each group and build from there.

Eating well is quite simple: "Eat food. Not too much. Mostly plants," as Michael Pollan put it in his book *In Defense of Food: An Eater's Manifesto.*

Eating with the 2211 plan is simple to do on a meal-by-meal, day-by-day, and week-by-week basis. Everyone can adopt this eating pattern because it's so flexible and simple. What's even better, the 2211 EAT plan takes the science of what to eat and the research behind optimal eating and makes it simple for everyone.

We are bombarded by food marketing and food and nutrition influencers on social media that may offer quick fixes. We have so many choices to eat tasty foods with plenty of fat and sugar to keep us wanting more. And it can be confusing trying to figure out what to eat when we see food claims (regulated by the US government) and dietary supplement claims (not regulated by the US government) at every turn. Reading food labels can also be confusing. So let's simplify food choices to make it easy to eat well and feel good about it.

What the Research Says

The 2211 EAT plan is reinforced by decades of research findings for health and well-being from eating a Mediterranean-type diet, the DASH (Dietary Approaches to Stop Hypertension) diet, and the MIND (Mediterranean-DASH Intervention for Neuro-degenerative Delay) diet. All three of these diets encourage eating a plant-based diet with ample fruits and vegetables, whole grains, healthy fats, and lean proteins.

We also have EAT recommendations based on solid science from large health organizations, including the American Heart Association and the American Cancer Society. In addition, we also get guidance from the Dietary Guidelines for Americans, put out by the federal government, which are updated every five years.

All these guidelines provide a framework for eating based on current science. The National Center for Complementary and Integrative Health also provides research-based guidelines for health and well-being.

With EAT MOVE GROOVE, these guidelines and recommendations are blended with practical, positive tips to support an EAT program that has these key choices as a foundation:

- Choose a plant-forward eating plan to optimize health and well-being.

- Eat a wide range of fruits and vegetables every day (at least 6 cups).
- Eat whole foods whenever possible, especially fruits, vegetables, and whole grains.
- Include protein-rich foods in every meal and snack.
- Choose healthy fats each day.
- Eat in moderation, listening to your body.
- Focus on what to eat instead of what not to eat.
- Enjoy your food!

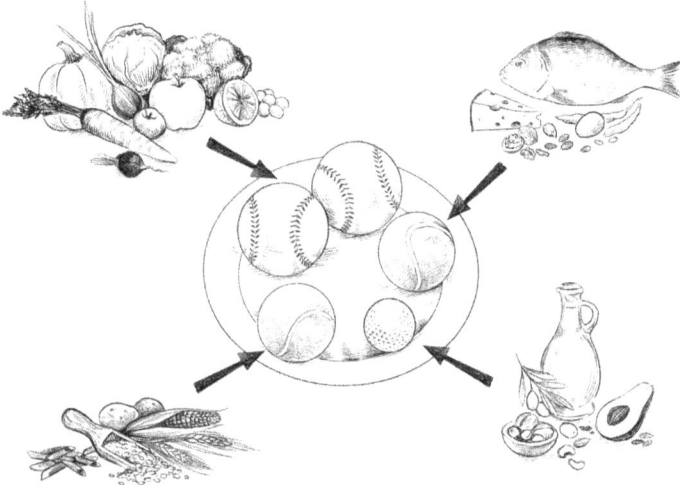

Produce, Protein, Grain, and Healthy Fat Serving Options

EAT Food Servings

Let's take a closer look at how the food groups (produce, protein, grains, and healthy fats) are easily set up in the 2211 plan. We'll begin with the superfoods of the plan: produce.

Produce

Thousands of research studies from all over the world reinforce the health benefits of eating fruits and vegetables and compounds found in these foods. Results from a 2021 study following nurses and health professionals in the US found that eating five cups of fruits and vegetables a day resulted in the greatest longevity.

In a study published several years earlier exploring the food intake of over 65,000 people in England, eating more fruits and vegetables (especially vegetables) was associated with better health outcomes and longevity. The more fruits and vegetables eaten, the better. Eating as many as seven servings or more a day of fruit and vegetables was the most beneficial for health. To be even more specific, the greatest health benefit was seen with high consumption of fresh vegetables, salads, fresh fruit, and dried fruit.

In another large study with over 450,000 people across ten countries, for every 2 cups of fruits and vegetables consumed each day, people lived longer.

Quite simply, eating more produce boosts our chances of having a longer life and staying healthy as we age.

Studies continue to demonstrate that eating a plant-based diet (plenty of fruits, vegetables, and whole grains) enhances health and well-being. In fact, a 2022 study comparing diets of over 10,000 people found that the risk of developing type 2 diabetes was lower if participants followed a plant-based diet including ample fruits, vegetables, nuts, legumes, and coffee. The researchers noted that their findings support the beneficial role of including healthy plant-based diets in diabetes prevention.

Plant-Forward Eating Is Good for the Planet

Eating more fruits and vegetables is so good for us from a health standpoint. But there's another critical reason the 2211 plan recommends 2 cups of produce at each meal. This is also very good for the planet. According to the EAT-Lancet Commission, a report from thirty-seven leading scientists from sixteen countries around the world defining targets for healthy diets for sustainable food production, a diet rich in plant-based foods and lower in animal foods can improve health and have positive effects on the environment.

Eating more fruits and vegetables is especially helpful if you want to enhance your health and boost the health of the planet at the same time.

The EAT-Lancet Commission report recommends eating approximately 2 cups of fruit and 3 cups of vegetables a day. The 2211 plan meets and even exceeds these recommendations by having 6 cups of produce a day.

Despite all we know about the benefits of eating more produce, according to the Produce for Better Health Foundation, our produce consumption continues to decrease in the US. In fact, according to the Centers for Disease Control and Prevention, only one in ten Americans is currently meeting fruit and vegetable intake recommendations.

You can find a myriad of great ideas for eating more fruits and vegetables with recipes and tips at *fruitsandveggies.org*.

"When it comes to eating produce, there are lots of ways to maximize the wealth on your shelf," says Leslie Bonci, MPH, RD, CSSD, Registered Dietitian and owner of Active Eating Advice by Leslie Bonci Inc. "Think about ways to enhance, embellish, and increase produce intake—add produce to mac and cheese, noodle dishes, use pasta sauce and tomato sauce in dishes, and add dried fruit like raisins to salads."

Here's the bottom line from these studies (and many others):

- Eat enough fruits and vegetables a day—6+ cups a day in the **2211** plan *meets or exceeds* the amounts consumed in most studies.

- Include plenty of fresh fruits and vegetables in your daily food choices when available.

- Choose local produce when you can. When produce is picked fresh, it's much higher in nutrients than produce that must travel a long way to get to you.

- Frozen fruits and vegetables are picked fresh and flash frozen, so they retain high levels of nutrients. Plus, you can easily find them without added sugar or salt.

- Try canned fruits and vegetables too. Look for fruit canned in water or its own juice and choose low salt or no added salt canned vegetables.

- Choose organically grown produce if it fits in your budget. Often, locally grown produce is also organically grown. In the stores, organically grown produce may be reasonably priced if it's in season.

- Eat produce that's in season. I get so much joy out of eating a delicious variety of produce as the availability of fruits and vegetables changes throughout the year based on growing seasons. Add variety to your produce intake by staying in tune to seasonal options.

- Prioritize eating vegetables in addition to fruits. Vegetables provide more health protection than fruits, so include them (especially raw vegetables) whenever possible.

- Frozen, canned, dried, sauces, juices, jars, and soups are all beneficial. Choose options that work with your tastes and budget.

22 Produce Picks for Your Grocery Cart

- **Fresh:** avocados, bananas, apples, grapes, broccoli, carrots, dark green leafy lettuce, tomatoes, spinach, onions, potatoes, peppers
- **Frozen:** mixed berries, mixed veggies
- **Canned:** peaches, pumpkin
- **Dried:** apricots, 100% fruit bars
- **Juices:** 100% fruit juices, 100% vegetable juices
- **Jars:** salsa, pasta sauce

Eat the Rainbow

Perhaps you've heard the recommendation to eat the rainbow when it comes to choosing fruits and vegetables. There's a good reason for this.

The nutrients in produce are visible to us by looking at the colors of fruits and vegetables. Fruits and vegetables contain vitamins, minerals, fiber, and other compounds, such as antioxidants and flavonoids, that provide protective health benefits when we eat them.

These food components give fruits and vegetables their vibrant colors. When you see and eat many different colors of fruits and vegetables on your plate, you reap the benefit of a wide range of nutrients. More color equals more nutrients. It's that simple.

Choosing Produce at the Market

Whether you're buying your produce from a grocery store or from a farmers' market, choosing the freshest produce possible has many benefits. First, when produce is fresh, it's generally been picked more recently. Second, fresh produce can be higher in nutrients than fruits and vegetables that have been sitting on the shelves for days or weeks. Third, fresh produce tastes better. When it tastes better, we eat more of it.

Here's what to look for:

- Choose fresh fruits and vegetables that don't have bruises, blemishes, cuts, wrinkles, or dark or soft spots. Inspect produce sold in bags closely by viewing the entire bag's contents.

- Look for vibrant colors. The color of produce gives you a hint about its nutritional value. More color often means higher nutrients.

- Buy small fruits and veggies if you want a burst of flavor. Many times, the smaller the fruit, the stronger the flavor. Think grape tomatoes, mini potatoes, or sweet cherries.

- Be gentle with fruits and veggies. Avoid bruising when you put your produce in the cart, bag your groceries, carry them, and put away your produce at home.

- When possible, seek out local farmers' markets to find produce at its peak. You can't beat local produce that's been recently harvested for freshness, flavor, and nutrition. Local, farmer-grown produce is often organically grown as well.

- Grow your own produce. You might have a garden space in your yard, rent a space in your community, or even start an herb garden in pots on your patio.

- Produce can look funny, have odd shapes, and still be perfectly ripe and highly nutritious. Treat yourself to some interesting-looking produce every now and then.

FEAR NOT THE FUNNY LOOKING FRUITS AND VEGGIES

According to Feeding America, nearly 40% of all food in the United States goes to waste. Much of that food comes directly from our kitchens. Whether you bring home produce that's not as fresh as you expected, or you find your fruits or veggies are going bad in the fridge, there are ways to get the most out of your produce and avoid wasting these fruits and veggies and save you money. Here's how:

- Make a big pot of vegetable soup or stew with veggies before you throw them out. Many times, you can save some parts of the produce (for example, the half of a green pepper that is still good), chop it up, and use in a soup or stew.

- Before throwing out those brown bananas, cut them into slices, freeze on a cookie sheet, and place in a sealed container or baggie in the freezer. Add to smoothies, banana bread, or muffins at a later time.

- Berries or peaches going soft? Rinse them well, freeze in an airtight container or baggie, and use in a smoothie, cobbler, or muffins.

- Blend fruit that's beginning to over-ripen (berries, melon, peaches, plums, mangos, or grapes), mix with yogurt, and pour into popsicle molds for a fruity frozen treat.

- Add layers of flavor. Sauté chopped greens, onions, peppers, tomatoes, zucchini, and carrots together with garlic, cook down and add layers of goodness to lasagna, pasta bakes, or shepherd's pie.

- Make a veggie frittata for breakfast, lunch, or dinner. Try the simple veggie frittata recipe in this book as a way to use up veggies such as greens, spinach, tomatoes, peppers, and even cooked potatoes, sweet potatoes, and onions.

Broaden Your Color Spectrum: Try These Fruits and Veggies

Red: cherries, tomatoes, beets, strawberries, raspberries, plums, grapefruit, red apples, lychee, red peppers, radishes, red lettuce, radicchio, red leaf lettuce, red cabbage, red grapes, pomegranates, guava, cranberries, goji berries, and red onions

Orange and yellow: carrots, mangos, papayas, apricots, peaches, nectarines, orange and yellow peppers, orange beets, oranges, tangerines, lemons, acorn squash, butternut squash, and yellow squash

Green: collard greens, mustard greens, turnip greens, broccoli, kale, dark lettuce, arugula, spinach, bok choy, green beans, cucumbers, kiwifruit, green apples, grapes, brussels sprouts, cabbage, sprouts, zucchini, and limes

White and light green: onions, cauliflower, mushrooms, pears, garlic, leeks, watercress, celery, bananas, plantains, kohlrabi, bamboo shoots, Napa cabbage, endive, fennel, rutabaga, and turnips

Blue and purple: grapes, purple kale, plums, blueberries, blackberries, eggplant, purple asparagus, purple potatoes, purple cabbage, and purple carrots

Take Inventory

Take a few minutes to investigate all the fruits and vegetables you have on hand now. Check for produce in fresh, frozen, canned, dried, freeze-dried, 100% juices, and sauces. Make a list of all the fruits and vegetables you currently have according to color. This will help you plan your grocery list later. Write your list on a piece of paper, note the list in your phone, or use the free downloadable Kitchen Inventory Sheet at *eatmovegroove.com.*

Once you've made a list of the foods you have on hand from each serving group, you can make a grocery list to add items to each serving group.

Proteins

With the simple **22**11 lifestyle plan, the eating plan prioritizes eating produce and protein in your meals. You'll eat 2 cups of produce and at least 2 ounces of protein in every meal. That's your **22** in the **22**11 plan. There's no question that fruits and vegetables come in front and center in a health-enhancing eating plan. Eating protein at meals and snacks has many benefits as well. With the **22**11 plan, you will eat at least 2 ounces (15 grams) of protein per meal.

What Is 2 Ounces of Protein?

When checking out the Nutrition Facts on a food package label, 2 ounces of protein is equal to about 15 grams of protein. When tracking your protein, either amount is equal to one protein serving.

To give you an idea of portion sizes, 2 ounces of protein is about 1 cup of cooked beans, ½ cup of nuts, 2 eggs, or 2 cups of milk or soy milk.

For high-protein animal foods such as beef, pork, chicken, or fish, a 2-ounce (weight) cooked portion is a serving. That's a little less than the size of a deck of cards. All these servings equal about 15 grams of protein on the food label.

Protein Supports Our Bodies

When we eat protein, we fuel our muscles and our tissues. Protein strengthens our body. This is critical. When we maintain our muscles, bones, and other bodily tissues, we can do more. It's that simple. Feed your body, and your body can better move you. As we age, this is even more important to maintain strength (along with doing strengthening exercises) and lower the risk of injuries and falls.

The simple 2211 lifestyle plan is set up so that protein-rich foods are eaten at every meal (and snacks). Typically, many people eat very little protein at breakfast, a little more protein at lunch, and then load up on protein at the evening meal. Simply being mindful to include at least 2 ounces of protein at breakfast can help your body stay strong. Essentially, you are telling your body that you have protein coming on board right away each day to help fuel and repair your muscles and tissues.

Some protein is found in other foods, too, such as whole grains, vegetables, and even in many of your love foods, so your total protein intake from a meal will be more than the 2 ounces of protein you get from your protein foods. That's great. While we don't need to go overboard, it's essential to consume some protein at every meal. For some meals, you may eat 3 or 4 ounces of protein in total. That works too.

Include Protein in Snacks

With the 2211 plan, you may choose to eat one or two snacks a day in addition to your meals if you get hungry between meals. To maximize the nutrition in your snacks (and your body), mix 1 cup of produce with 1 ounce of protein (around 7 grams on the Nutrition Facts label). Try a handful of mixed nuts with an apple if you're on the go. Or blend up a quick smoothie with ½ cup frozen berries, ½ cup orange juice, and ½ cup Greek yogurt.

Adding one to two snacks a day with protein can boost protein intake by another 7 to 15 grams a day and can provide an additional way to optimize daily protein intake. And if you prefer not to eat snacks, you will be meeting your protein needs either way.

Figuring Your Daily Protein Needs

Total protein daily recommendations are based on body weight (more specifically, lean muscle mass), age, and activity. Your total protein intake with the 2211 plan will vary depending on the specific foods you eat, which foods you choose to add for your love foods, whether you add snacks to your daily intake, and the types of grains and vegetables you choose.

Based on a diet analysis from consumers who follow the 2211 plan, typical protein intake averages between 70 to 100 grams of protein a day from meals and snacks.

An easy way to determine your minimum personal daily protein needs is to follow this simple recommendation:

1. Take your weight in pounds.
2. Divide your weight by 2. This is an estimate of your daily protein needs in grams.
3. Divide that number by 3 for 3 meals a day. This is an estimate of your recommended protein intake for each meal.

Let's look at a few examples:

1. Weight = 200 pounds
2. 200 pounds divided by 2 = 100. Daily protein needs are approximately 100 grams per day.
3. Protein intake per meal = 100 grams of protein divided by 3 meals per day = approximately 34 grams of protein per meal.

1. Weight = 150 pounds
2. 150 pounds divided by 2 = 75. Total daily protein needs = approximately 75 grams per day.
3. Protein intake per meal = 75 grams of protein divided by 3 meals per day = approximately 25 grams of protein per meal.

How to Read a Nutrition Facts Label

Eating protein at meals and snacks also helps us feel satisfied. We don't get hungry as fast after eating when we include foods high in protein. As an example, when we eat toast, fruit, or a bagel for breakfast, we digest these foods quickly. When you add high-protein foods like yogurt, peanut butter, or eggs, the meal takes longer to digest. If we feel more satisfied after eating, we tend to eat less overall. So if maintaining your weight or losing weight are included in your whys, this can be a big help.

High-protein plant-based foods and animal-based foods can both provide high-quality protein. If you choose to eat a meat-free diet or choose to cut back on animal-based foods, you can easily meet your protein needs with only plant-based foods.

So where's the protein? Check out the examples of 2 ounces of protein in the following foods (about 15 grams of protein on a Nutrition Facts label):

- 2 eggs
- 1 egg + 2 egg whites
- 2 cups of skim, 1%, or 2% milk
- 2 cups of soy milk, pea protein milk, or high-protein almond milk
- ¾ cup Greek yogurt
- 1 cup soy yogurt
- 1 ½ cups almond milk yogurt
- 2 ounces cheese (cheddar, Swiss, Parmesan)
- ¾ cup cottage cheese
- 3 mozzarella cheese sticks
- ½ cup shredded cheese (cheddar, Swiss, Parmesan)
- ½ cup nuts (peanuts, walnuts, almonds)
- ¼ cup peanut butter (or other nut butters)
- ½ cup sunflower seeds
- ½ cup pumpkin seeds
- ⅓ cup hemp seeds
- ¾ cup edamame (soybeans)
- ½ cup tofu
- ½ cup tempeh
- 1 to 2 veggie burger patties
- 1 cup cooked beans or legumes (black beans, kidney beans, white beans, lentils)
- ¾ cup hummus
- 2 ounces lean chicken breast (or ½ cup chopped)
- 2 ounces lean beef sirloin (or ½ cup chopped)
- 2 ounces lean pork loin (or ½ cup chopped)
- 2 ounces fish (or ½ cup chopped)
- ¼ cup packed canned tuna or salmon
- 2 ounces ground turkey or ground lean beef (or ½ cup cooked)

To find the amount (grams) of protein in a food product on a Nutrition Facts label, look for Protein and check out the grams of protein per serving. In the case of this Easy Turkey & Veggie Chili recipe, one serving has 19.4 grams of protein. Since 2 ounces of protein is about 15 grams of protein, this food provides about 2½ ounces of protein per serving.

Easy Turkey & Veggie Chili		
Nutrition Facts		
Serving Size		1 Serving
Amount Per Serving		
Calories		**247.4**
		% Daily Value*
Total Fat	6.2 g	8 %
Saturated Fat	1.5 g	8 %
Trans Fat	0.1 g	
Cholesterol	47.2 mg	16 %
Sodium	757.7 mg	33 %
Total Carbohydrate	30.9 g	11 %
Dietary Fiber	9.4 g	33 %
Total Sugars	4.9 g	
Added Sugars	0 g	0 %
Protein	19.4 g	
Vitamin D	0.1 mcg	0 %
Calcium	68.5 mg	5 %
Iron	3 mg	17 %
Potassium	803 mg	17 %

* The % Daily Value (DV) tells you how much a nutrient in a serving of food contributes to a daily diet. 2,000 calories a day is used for general nutrition advice.

Full Info at cronometer.com   </>

Take Inventory

Take a few minutes to investigate all the protein-rich foods you currently have at home. Check for proteins in the refrigerator, freezer, and pantry. As with your produce, check the foods you have on hand to write your grocery lists later. Add proteins to your Kitchen Inventory Sheet at *eatmovegroove.com.*

Grains and Starches

In the simple 2211 lifestyle plan, the first 1 equals grain or starch. Grains (especially whole grains) provide important nutrients such as carbohydrates, fiber, vitamins, and minerals to your body. In the 2211 plan, you choose any grains you like. When possible, eat whole grains, as they offer a big nutrition boost and are a great source of fiber.

Whole Grains Explained

According to the Whole Grains Council, whole grains or foods made from them contain all the essential parts and naturally occurring nutrients of the entire grain seed in their original proportions. Simply put, when you eat whole grains, you eat the whole grain—the whole thing. For example, when you eat 100 percent whole-wheat bread, you eat bread with flour made from whole wheat kernels. If you purchase a product that simply says "bread," then you may be eating only part of the grain. What is usually stripped away is the good stuff like the fiber, vitamins, and minerals.

Whole grains contain all three parts of the original grain: the bran (outer skin of the grain), the germ (or the embryo of the plant that can sprout into a new plant), and the endosperm (the grain's food supply, made mostly of starch). When grains are missing at least one part, they are no longer considered whole grains. Examples of refined grains are white rice and white flour, both with their bran and germ removed. They still provide some nutrients, but not nearly as many as the whole grain.

Reasons to Eat Whole Grains

First, whole grains offer more nutrients than refined grains (grains that are processed and broken down, so they don't include the whole part of the grains). Whole grains provide more fiber, vitamins, minerals, protein, healthy fats, and antioxidants.

Second, a large amount of sound, decades-old scientific evidence shows that eating whole grains can lower your risk of developing heart disease, stroke, diabetes, and certain cancers. Replacing refined grains with whole grains can help lower blood sugar and blood pressure and can even help keep your weight in check.

Third, more whole-grain consumption and more dietary fiber consumption are both associated with a longer lifespan. One large review investigated over 200 studies on whole grain and fiber consumption. A high intake of whole grains and fiber (instead of refined grains) was correlated with a 15 to 30 percent increase in longevity. That's worth every kernel.

It's not difficult to choose whole grains over refined grains most of the time. That's not to say you can't have your favorite refined grains. For example, you may love white rice. It's still good for you, so enjoy it, but also try brown rice. You may surprise yourself and love the hearty texture. You may love white sourdough bread. While most sourdough bread is made from refined grain (the outer part of the wheat berry has been removed), sourdough bread can still fit in the plan as not every grain serving you eat needs to be 100% whole grain. But for an extra nutrition punch, try whole-wheat sourdough bread. You can also try substituting whole-grain pasta for regular pasta.

You may have your favorite refined grains, but I encourage you to try some new whole grains. You will be pleasantly surprised by what you find. There are many options to choose from, as the following list shows. When these grains or grain flours contain the three parts of the whole grain (bran, germ, and endosperm), they are considered whole grains. For more information, tips for using these grains, and recipes, check out the Whole Grains Council at *wholegrainscouncil.org*.

Whole Grains

Whole grains contain the entire grain and are great options to boost your nutrition. Try these whole grains in your **2211** EAT plan.

- Corn
- Rice
- Wild rice
- Wheat
- Oats
- Barley
- Popcorn
- Rye
- Spelt
- Sorghum
- Quinoa
- Amaranth
- Buckwheat
- Millet
- Teff
- Triticale
- Emmer
- Farro

Starchy Vegetables

In the **2211** plan, the 1 for grains also includes eating starchy vegetables as an option. Why are starchy vegetables included in the grain area? Nutritionally, many starchy vegetables are much more in line with grains than vegetables when comparing nutritional value. For example, starchy vegetables such as potatoes and peas have a greater amount of carbohydrate (and more calories) than most vegetables.

Starchy vegetables include the following foods:

- Potatoes
- Sweet potatoes
- Purple potatoes
- Yams
- Pumpkin
- Butternut squash
- Acorn squash
- Peas
- Cassava
- Parsnips
- Taro

Take Inventory

Take a few minutes to investigate all the grains and starches you currently have on hand and add them to your Kitchen Inventory Sheet.

You may find them in the pantry, in the refrigerator, in the freezer, or on your counter. You may have both whole grains and refined grains. Many grain-based foods we purchase in the grocery store are refined grains. Moving toward eating more whole grains can take some time and practice. Try them and see what you like.

Try purchasing more starchy vegetables as well. Once you make a list of what you currently have on hand, you can add more whole grains and starchy vegetables to your list to download at *eatmovegroove.com.*

Healthy Fats

The final 1 in the **2211** EAT plan refers to healthy fats. We need fat for overall health, so it's important to choose fats that are good for you. With the **2211** plan, you'll choose healthy fats or super fats to eat most often. Most of the time, choose these healthy fats. These foods can boost your health while providing essential nutrients like vitamins A, D, and E. Of course, you may occasionally enjoy fats like butter, deep-fried foods, or flavorful coconut oil in a dish.

By choosing healthy fat sources in small amounts with each meal, you optimize the health benefits of eating fats, but don't eat too much fat. For most people, it's best to keep total fat intake to 30 percent of the total diet. This equals about 500 to 600 calories (or 55 to 67 grams of fat) in a 1,600 to 2,000 calorie plan. When looking at a Nutrition Facts label, 5 grams of fat equals about 50 calories. That's the amount of fat in one teaspoon of oil.

HEALTHY FATS EXPLAINED

In the EAT MOVE GROOVE **22**11 program, you eat healthy fats that are high in monounsaturated, polyunsaturated, and omega-3 fatty acids. Saturated fats (generally fats that are hard at room temperature) and trans fats (similar fats made from oils that can raise blood cholesterol) are the kinds of fats we want to keep to a minimum for overall health.

What are the fats we want to eat more of, what do they do for your health, and which foods are good sources?

Monounsaturated fats can help reduce low-density lipoprotein (LDL), or "bad" cholesterol levels and decrease your risk for developing heart disease. Common sources: olive oil, avocado oil, canola oil, peanut oil, safflower oil, sesame oil, avocados, eggs, nuts, seeds, and nut butters.

Polyunsaturated fats can also help reduce LDL cholesterol levels and decrease your risk for developing heart disease. Common sources: soybean oil, corn oil, sunflower oil, nuts, and flaxseeds.

Omega-3 fatty acids are a family of polyunsaturated fatty acids that enhance health by lowering LDL and total cholesterol levels. Common sources: fatty fish such as tuna, salmon, sardines, mackerel, and trout; fish oil, flaxseed oil, flaxseeds, chia seeds, walnuts, and omega-3 fortified eggs.

Foods with Healthy Fats

Choose the following foods often for your healthy fats. These foods are high in monounsaturated, polyunsaturated, and/or omega-3 fatty acids, so they are good for you.

"Look for ways to add healthy fats to foods you already eat during the day," says Registered Dietitian Lisa Burgoon. She suggests adding nuts, seeds, and avocados to everything from oatmeal to salads to boost healthy fats and help manage health concerns like high cholesterol naturally.

- **Avocados:** Avocados are a great source of healthy monounsaturated fats and are also high in fiber. Slice half of an avocado to add to any meal and you'll be on the right track with the **2211** plan.

- **Olives:** An integral part of the Mediterranean diet, olives are a fantastic staple in the **2211** plan. Add 2 Tablespoons, or a small handful, of olives to your meal to boost the healthy fat content and provide a burst of flavor too.

- **Oils:** Choose vegetable oils high in monounsaturated and polyunsaturated fats as your primary oils, including olive oil, avocado oil, canola oil, peanut oil, safflower oil, flaxseed oil, corn oil, soybean oil, and sunflower oil. Add a tablespoon to veggies when roasting or when cooking.

- **Salad dressings:** Choose salad dressing made with the oils above, including vinaigrettes, clear dressings like Italian dressing, and oil and vinegar dressings. Add a tablespoon of an oil-based dressing to salads.

Some foods are high in protein *and* healthy fats. These are great options for meals and snacks as you can eat 2+ ounces of protein and get your healthy fat in one food. Examples of these foods include the following:

- **Fatty fish:** Fish such as salmon, tuna, sardines, trout, herring, and mackerel contain omega-3 fatty acids, which are good for the body. They help maintain heart health. In fact, the American Heart Association recommends eating two 3-ounce servings of fatty fish a week to boost heart health.

- **Eggs:** The yolk of the egg is an excellent source of fat, while whole eggs are a great protein option. Not only does an egg yolk contain a mix of different kinds of fats (monounsaturated, saturated, and polyunsaturated), it's also a good source of vitamin D and choline, a vitamin-like substance that supports a healthy heart. The vibrant color of the egg yolk is also a reminder that egg yolks have high amounts of antioxidants, which promote health. You can also purchase omega-3 fortified eggs.

- **Nuts:** Eat a handful of nuts every day. That's about ¼ cup of nuts, providing one ounce of protein and a healthy dose of health-promoting fats too. Or eat 2 Tablespoons of nut butter. Many studies have highlighted the health benefits of eating nuts daily, including lowering cholesterol, decreasing inflammation, and lowering the risk of developing heart disease and certain cancers. What's not to love?

- **Nut and seed butters:** Spreading health is so easy with peanut butter, almond butter, walnut butter, pistachio butter—the list goes on. You can choose your favorites in the grocery store and find natural varieties without added salt or sugar. Adding 2 Tablespoons to a meal offers 1 ounce of protein and healthy fats.

- **Chia seeds:** Tiny chia seeds are a great plant source of health-promoting omega-3 fatty acids. They are also high in many other nutrients, including fiber, iron, and antioxidants. Sprinkle a tablespoon of chia seeds on yogurt or in your salad.

- **Ground flaxseeds (flaxseed meal):** Flaxseeds are also high in fiber and omega-3 fatty acids. Eat ground flaxseeds to get the full benefit of these seeds. Add a tablespoon to oatmeal in the morning for a nutty flavor.

- **Hemp seeds:** Hemp seeds are small brown seeds that are high in protein and healthy fats and boast a nutty, earthy flavor. You can eat the whole seed or the soft hemp hearts with the shell removed. Add 3 Tablespoons to a meal, and you get over an ounce of protein, along with a boost of omega-3 fatty acids and magnesium.

Take Inventory

Take inventory of the healthy fats you have on hand now. Check your pantry, refrigerator, freezer, and counter. Add these healthy fats to your Kitchen Inventory Sheet at *eatmovegroove.com.*

Love Foods

Include a love food (a food you just want to eat because you love it) once or twice a day with the **2211** plan if you prefer. Why? First, it's wonderful to delight in our food. We eat food, not just nutrients. Food is to be enjoyed. That may sound odd coming from a Registered Dietitian, but it's true. Again, I will repeat: **Food is to be enjoyed.**

When you include foods you simply love to eat every day, you feel good about what you're eating. That's essential when building and maintaining the EAT MOVE GROOVE lifestyle. With the **2211** plan, include foods that help you groove, or feel good about yourself. There is no guilt with **2211**. We can still be mindful of what we are eating and how much we are eating and, at the same time, enjoy all foods.

I grew up in a big family where we got used to having a little something sweet after dinner every night. It was often a low-cost dessert like cake made from a boxed mix, a few cookies, a handful of chocolate stars, or a scoop of ice cream. Suffice it to say that in my childhood home, dessert was something we anticipated after meals, and we enjoyed it.

To this day, if I feel like it, I enjoy having a little something sweet after meals. It makes me feel like the meal is complete and I can move on to whatever is coming next in my day. You may have similar experiences, or you may enjoy a cocktail or a glass of wine with dinner. Maybe you love salty snacks. You may have other favorite foods you simply love to eat. There's room for your favorites with the 2211 plan.

When we're flexible with our eating, and when we're mindful of eating in moderation, no foods are off limits. This supportive thinking allows for more positivity with our eating, and, in turn, we can also treat our bodies and nurture them. If foods are not forbidden, we have the freedom to enjoy them in smaller amounts and know they are available to us at any time. Think about it. Taking away the "shoulds" allows us the liberty to eat foods that fuel us nutritionally and fuel us psychologically and emotionally too.

How many times have you said to yourself, "I know I'm full, but I still want that dessert because it looks so good." Give yourself a moment to reflect. Maybe you really don't want dessert. Or maybe enjoying a small portion of the dessert can satisfy you because you know it's not forbidden to you. We don't need to eat a pint of ice cream when we know we could eat ice cream every day. This thinking takes away the power of that food and helps us enjoy the pleasure of eating. I encourage you to enjoy your love foods. Take time to eat them and be sure to savor them.

Sometimes you'll feel satisfied without adding a love food to your meal. Other times, you may really enjoy having something you just crave. You can choose how you employ the love foods with the 2211 plan. They are built into the day, so you know they are an option to you every day.

With the **2211** simple EAT plan, love foods can be included in any meal or snack in the day. The caveat is to be mindful of the amount of love foods you're eating. Plan out your love foods to around 100-calorie portions. This offers an opportunity to enjoy your favorite foods in moderation, or in smaller amounts. Sometimes we feel more satisfied if we "eat the whole thing." Because of this, finishing off a portion of a love food, even if it's small, may be enough to enjoy your treat, but not overdo it, keeping the total calories in the plan lower.

Here are some options you may enjoy for love foods. Add one or two foods you like in a day, being mindful of the portion or amount of food that equates to about 100 calories.

Love Foods with around 100 Calories

- Mini ice cream bars
- Mini frozen yogurt bars
- Frozen chocolate-covered banana slices
- Snack-size pudding cups
- Single-serving 100-calorie cookie packs
- Single-serving 100-calorie pretzel or chips bags
- Single-serving 100-calorie granola bars
- 1 ounce of dark chocolate
- 4 chocolate stars
- 4 chocolate kisses
- 1 dark chocolate caramel square
- Handful of chocolate-covered almonds
- Handful of potato chips
- Handful of pretzels
- 1 ounce small box of sugared cereal
- Snack-size candy bars
- 2 graham cracker squares
- 1 ounce of dark chocolate
- 1 ounce of hard candy

- 5 ounces of wine
- 12 ounces of lite beer
- 1 ounce of hard liquor

Action Steps

The **2211** EAT recommendations are simple and easy to put into action.

- Eat a plant-forward diet (mostly fruits, vegetables, and whole grains).
- Include 2 cups of produce as part of every meal.
- Include 2 or more ounces of plant- or animal-based protein with every meal. It's your choice. Try plant-based proteins even if you're a meat eater.
- Eat 1 grain or starch with every meal (especially whole grains).
- Enjoy healthy fats with every meal.
- Try new foods and food combinations. You may be surprised by what you enjoy. Explore flavorful herbs and spices to enhance your eating experience.

You'll find foods to build your personal **2211** around in the next chapter. Come back to your why and take note of foods that will provide you with targeted benefits every day.

4

Foods to Fuel Your Why

E AT MOVE GROOVE may resonate with you because you're interested in maintaining your health in a proactive way. Or you may have health concerns managed in part by eating a specific diet or adding prescriptive foods. Perhaps you know you're at risk for certain health concerns based on your genetics or family history and you want to find foods that will help lower your risk.

In addition to utilizing the 2211 plan to help manage your whys, and if you need more personalized guidance, it's a good idea to work with your healthcare team to be sure you are eating to help manage your specific health concerns. For nutrition recommendations tailored to your individual medical needs, meet with a Registered Dietitian Nutritionist (RD/RDN), an expert with comprehensive training in how the foods you eat impact your health. You can find a nutrition expert near you on the Academy of Nutrition and Dietetics website at *eatright.org*.

Because the EAT MOVE GROOVE plan is so flexible, it meets the needs of many of the most common health concerns such as hypertension (high blood pressure), high cholesterol, and arthritis. You can tweak the plan to focus on the foods that are of greatest benefit to you. You'll find lists of foods to include more often based on common health and wellness goals and several common health concerns.

Remember that all fruits and vegetables are excellent choices, as well as lean proteins, whole grains, and healthy fats. These lists may spark new ideas for adding foods you've gotten away from. The biggest benefit you will receive is eating the 2211 way, and trying new foods.

Eating for Heart Health

Like the 2211 EAT plan, the American Heart Association (AHA) recommends eating a wide variety of fruits and vegetables, whole grains, healthy sources of protein such as beans, nuts, fish, low-fat dairy foods, lean meats, and healthy fats. The AHA also suggests minimizing the intake of added sugars, being mindful of salt intake, and going easy with alcohol or avoiding it altogether. There are specific foods you can eat more often that help with lowering cholesterol or managing blood pressure if these are concerns for you. These are smart foods for everyone, but they may be even more beneficial if heart health is one of your whys.

What to Eat to Lower Cholesterol and Boost Heart Health

All fruits and veggies are healthy options to boost heart health. Eat more produce daily to lower your risk of developing heart disease. Include all fruits and vegetables you enjoy. Eat more dried beans and peas as they contain gooey or gummy fibers that can help lower total and LDL blood cholesterol levels. Choose more avocados, whole grains, nuts, seeds, and fatty fish from this list of foods to lower cholesterol.

Produce

- Apples
- Berries, including blueberries, blackberries, strawberries, raspberries, and others
- Broccoli
- Citrus fruits, including oranges, grapefruit, and tangerines
- Dark greens, including spinach, kale, arugula, bok choy, collards, dandelion greens, Swiss chard, and mustard greens (fresh or frozen)
- Eggplant
- Okra
- Pears
- Tomatoes, including fresh, canned, sauces, and salsa

Proteins

- Beans and peas (legumes), including black beans, kidney beans, garbanzo beans, lentils, and others
- Eggs, especially high omega-3 eggs
- Fatty fish, especially salmon, tuna, sardines, and lake trout
- Nuts, especially walnuts, peanuts, cashews, almonds, macadamia nuts, pecans, hazelnuts, and nut butters
- Seeds, especially sunflower seeds, pumpkin seeds, ground flax seeds, chia seeds, hemp seeds, sesame seeds, and seed butters
- Soy-based foods, including edamame, tofu, tempeh, miso, soy yogurt, and soy milk

Grains and Starches

- Barley
- Brown rice

- Oats, including whole oats (oat groats), steel-cut oats, oat bran, old- fashioned oats, and quick oats
- Quinoa

Healthy Fats

- Avocados, guacamole, and avocado oil
- Eggs, especially high omega-3 eggs
- Fatty fish, especially salmon, tuna, sardines, and lake trout
- Nuts, especially walnuts, peanuts, cashews, almonds, macadamia nuts, pecans, hazelnuts, and nut butters
- Oils, especially extra virgin olive oil (EVOO), safflower oil, grapeseed oil, sesame oil, and canola oil
- Seeds, especially sunflower seeds, pumpkin seeds, ground flax seeds, chia seeds, hemp seeds, sesame seeds, and seed butters

Love Foods

- Dark chocolate, try a 1-ounce piece
- Red wine, enjoy a 5-ounce glass

Eating to Manage Blood Pressure

If managing high blood pressure is one of your whys, you can choose plenty of different foods to eat every day to help. If you are one of the nearly half of all Americans who have high blood pressure, eating more foods high in potassium, magnesium, calcium, and vitamin D can help keep your blood pressure in check. Too much sodium (salt) in the diet can cause too much water to go into the bloodstream and lead to high blood pressure in some people. On the other hand, eating foods high in potassium can lessen those effects and help manage high blood pressure.

Choose more of the foods in the following list to help lower blood pressure. Many of these foods to lower blood pressure are high in potassium, magnesium, calcium, or vitamin D.

Produce

- Bamboo shoots
- Bananas
- Carrots and carrot juice
- Coconut water
- Dark, leafy greens, especially beet greens, Swiss chard, and spinach (fresh or frozen)
- Dried apricots, dried peaches, and prunes
- Guava
- Jackfruit
- Kiwifruit
- Kohlrabi
- Melons, including cantaloupe, honeydew, and watermelon
- Onions
- Parsnips
- Plantains
- Portobello mushrooms
- Prune juice, apricot nectar, pomegranate juice, passionfruit juice, orange juice, pineapple juice, and tangerine juice
- Sapodilla
- Snow peas
- Tomatoes, tomato paste, tomato juice, tomato sauce, and salsa
- Water chestnuts

Proteins

- Beans and peas (legumes), especially lima beans, adzuki beans, white beans, black beans, and lentils
- Clams
- Fish, especially salmon, tuna, herring, sardines, trout, tilapia, shad, mullet, and pollock
- Hummus
- Milk, yogurt, kefir, and cheese
- Nuts and seeds, especially Brazil nuts, cashews, almonds, chia seeds, and pumpkin seeds
- Plant-based milks, including almond, oat, cashew, rice, and pea milks
- Soy-based foods including edamame, tofu, tempeh, miso, soy yogurt, and fortified soy milk

Grains and Starches

- Fufu (a West African dish)
- Squash, including acorn, butternut and spaghetti squash
- Sweet potatoes, purple potatoes, and yams
- Taro root
- White, yellow, and purple potatoes

Healthy Fats

- Avocados and avocado oil
- Fish, especially salmon, tuna, herring, sardines, trout, tilapia, shad, mullet, and pollock

Eating to Manage Prediabetes and Type 2 Diabetes

What you eat, how you move, and how you take care of your overall well-being can all enhance the management of prediabetes (higher than normal blood sugar, but not high enough to be considered type 2 diabetes) and diabetes. The foods you choose can help manage blood sugar levels.

According to the American Diabetes Association, good choices from food groups are those that are lower in saturated fat, trans fat, added sugars, and sodium (or salt) than similar foods in the same categories. Choosing foods with more fiber and protein can also be helpful with managing blood sugars. If you have prediabetes or diabetes, you can fine-tune the 2211 plan by working with your Registered Dietitian Nutritionist (RD/RDN) or your Certified Diabetes Care and Education Specialist (CDCES) to tailor it specifically to you.

For produce, choose fresh, frozen, and canned vegetables without added salt, and fresh, frozen, or canned fruits without added sugars. Milk, yogurt, and plant-based milks and milk products without added sugars are the best choices. Whole grains, beans, peas, plant-based proteins, fish, chicken, lean meats, and healthy fats are all recommended from this list of foods to help manage prediabetes and diabetes.

Produce

- Apples
- Asparagus
- Beets and beetroot juice
- Berries, including blueberries, blackberries, strawberries, raspberries, and others
- Broccoli
- Cabbage
- Cauliflower
- Cherries
- Citrus fruits, including oranges, grapefruit, and tangerines
- Dark, leafy greens, including romaine, Swiss chard, and spinach (fresh or frozen)

- Grapes
- Green beans
- Mushrooms
- Onions
- Peaches
- Pears
- Peppers
- Plums
- Tomatoes

Proteins

- Beans and peas (legumes), including black beans, kidney beans, garbanzo beans, lentils, and others
- Eggs
- Fat-free and low-fat milk
- Fish and shellfish, including cod, tilapia, salmon, tuna, shrimp, and crab
- Nuts, especially walnuts, peanuts, cashews, almonds, macadamia nuts, pecans, hazelnuts, and nut butters
- Plain, nonfat yogurt
- Seeds, especially sunflower seeds, pumpkin seeds, ground flax seeds, chia seeds, hemp seeds, sesame seeds, and seed butters
- Soy-based foods including edamame, tofu, tempeh, miso, and soy yogurt
- Unflavored soy milk and other plant-based milks

Grains and Starches

- Barley
- Bulgur
- Butternut squash and acorn squash
- Brown rice
- Corn and cornmeal

- Oats, including whole oats (oat groats), steel-cut oats, oat bran, old- fashioned oats, and quick oats
- Popcorn
- Pumpkin
- Sweet potatoes, purple potatoes, and yams
- Whole-grain cereal like wheat flakes, toasted oats, or rye flakes
- Whole-grain bread like whole wheat, rye, or oat
- Whole-grain breads

Healthy Fats

- Avocados, guacamole, and avocado oil
- Fish, especially salmon, tuna, herring, sardines, and lake trout
- Oils, especially extra virgin olive oil (EVOO), safflower oil, grapeseed oil, sesame oil, and canola oil
- Seeds, especially sunflower seeds, pumpkin seeds, ground flax seeds, chia seeds, hemp seeds, sesame seeds, and seed butters

Love Foods

- Dark chocolate, enjoy a 1-ounce piece

Eating to Manage Weight

If one of your goals is to eat to maintain or lose weight, choosing lower-calorie foods from each group will lower your calorie intake. Over weeks and months of time and combined with implementing the 2211 MOVE and GROOVE plan, you can support weight maintenance or weight loss.

Many factors affect weight changes. Choosing lower-calorie foods that also boost satiety, or a feeling of fullness and satisfaction, is one key to focus on. Simply eating more fruits and vegetables can help you lose weight by displacing higher-calorie foods in your diet. For example, by swapping a sliced apple for potato chips, you automatically cut down on your calorie intake. Put these foods for weight management on your grocery list and enjoy them often.

Produce

- Apples
- Berries, including blueberries, blackberries, strawberries, raspberries, and others
- Broccoli
- Brussels sprouts
- Cabbage, including red, green, and Napa
- Cauliflower
- Celery
- Cherries
- Citrus fruits, including oranges, grapefruit, and tangerines
- Cucumbers
- Dark greens, including spinach, kale, arugula, collards, bok choy, watercress, and Swiss chard (fresh or frozen)
- Dragon fruit
- Grapes
- Kiwifruit
- Melon, including watermelon, honeydew, and cantaloupe
- Mushrooms
- Onions
- Papaya
- Peaches
- Pears
- Peppers

- Pineapple
- Plums
- Pumpkin
- Radishes
- Sprouts, including alfalfa, mung bean, radish, broccoli, red clover, and wheatgrass
- Squash, including acorn, butternut and spaghetti squash
- Tomatoes

Protein

- Beans and peas (legumes), including black beans, kidney beans, garbanzo beans, lentils, and others
- Chicken breast and turkey breast (skinless)
- Edamame
- Eggs and egg whites
- Fish and shellfish. including cod, whitefish, tilapia, shrimp, lobster, mussels, oysters, scallops, and clams
- Lean meats, including beef sirloin, pork loin, and venison
- Mozzarella cheese and other low-fat cheeses
- Nonfat cottage cheese and nonfat ricotta cheese
- Nonfat or 1 percent milk
- Nonfat plant-based milks like soy milk, nut milks, pea milk, and oat milk
- Nonfat or 1 percent yogurt and Greek yogurt

Grains and Starches

- Barley
- Brown rice
- Corn
- Couscous

- Farro
- Potatoes and sweet potatoes
- Quinoa
- Whole-grain bread like whole wheat, rye, or oat
- Whole-grain cereal like wheat flakes, toasted oats, or rye flakes

Love Foods

Choose one to two love foods from the 100-calorie love foods list elsewhere in this book. Check portions and give yourself time to enjoy and savor your favorite love foods so you can feel satisfied with small amounts.

Anytime

- Green tea, black tea, and herbal teas
- Water flavored with slices of orange, lemon, and lime

HEALTHY FATS

Healthy fats are key components of an optimal diet and are included in all meals in the **22**11 plan. In fact, you must have some fat each day for good health. To help manage weight, include healthy fats such as olive oil and avocados in moderate amounts. While these foods contain good fats, they also add calories—1 gram of fat has 9 calories, while 1 gram of protein or carbohydrate has only 4 calories.

Including fats in small amounts will help you keep total calories down if weight management is one of your whys. Be aware of serving sizes. One teaspoon of oil contains about 50 calories. When cooking, start with 1 teaspoon of oil and add more if needed, being mindful of the extra calories. Similarly, go easy on salad dressings that contain oil, such as vinaigrette or Italian.

Two tablespoons of a fresh avocado (about 1/5 of an avocado or 3 slices) contains about 50 calories. This is a modest serving size, but avocado provides so many important nutrients to the diet, even in small amounts. If you love avocados, enjoy half of one at a meal. Just be aware that avocados are a higher-calorie food and modify your portions of the other foods in the meal if they are also high in calories.

Nuts and seeds are excellent sources of protein *and* healthy fats, but again, they are high in calories. I recommend measuring out nuts if you are being mindful of your calorie intake. For example, 2 Tablespoons of nuts is about 100 calories and 8 grams of fat, while 1 Tablespoon of peanut butter is also about 100 calories and 8 grams of fat. There are so many health benefits of eating nuts and seeds in moderation but be aware that calories can add up fast.

100 CALORIES OF NUTS

If you're watching your calorie intake, here's a quick guide to the average number of nuts in 100 calories:

Almonds: 14
Brazil nuts: 3
Cashews: 10
Hazelnuts: 10
Macadamia Nuts: 6
Peanuts: 16
Pecans: 10
Pistachios: 29
Walnuts: 9 halves

Eating to Maintain a Healthy Gut

One of the most important aspects of overall health is the health of the gastrointestinal tract, or the gut. Maintaining a healthy gut can help our bodies digest food better and keep the gut microbiome, or all the bacteria and microbes in your gut, in good working order. Keeping your gut healthy can have a positive impact on other parts of your body, including your brain, your heart, and your immune system. While we can't see inside the gut, we now know that "feeding" the body means feeding the gut with optimal foods.

Eating a high-fiber diet with plenty of fruits, vegetables, and whole grains is the cornerstone for maintaining gut health. Eating according to the 2211 lifestyle plan meets these recommendations. Some specific foods may provide additional benefits for gut health.

Prebiotic foods are high-fiber foods that support the beneficial bacteria in your gut, including bananas, oats, beans, and artichokes.

Probiotics are foods that naturally contain beneficial bacteria, including yogurt and fermented foods such as sauerkraut, pickles, kimchi, and kombucha.

Both prebiotics and probiotics help improve your digestion and keep your gut healthy. That's important for many reasons and may play key roles in overall health and well-being. Other foods help with digestion by boosting fiber or adding important nutrients. Choose these foods more often to support your gut health every day.

Produce

- Artichokes, especially Jerusalem artichokes
- Bananas
- Beets
- Berries, including blueberries, blackberries, strawberries, raspberries, and others
- Brussels sprouts
- Kimchi
- Leeks

- Miso vegetable soup
- Onions
- Sauerkraut

Proteins

- Beans and peas (legumes), including black beans, kidney beans, garbanzo beans, lentils, and others
- Fatty fish, including canned and fresh salmon, tuna, sardines, and lake trout
- Kefir
- Miso
- Natto (fermented soybeans)
- Nuts, including almonds, pine nuts, pecans, hazelnuts, and walnuts
- Seeds, including chia seeds, sunflower seeds, pumpkin seeds, and ground flax seeds
- Tempeh
- Yogurt with live cultures

Grains

- Brown rice
- Bulgur
- Oats, including whole oat groats, steel-cut oats, oat bran, old-fashioned oats, and quick oats
- Sourdough bread
- Whole wheat and wheat bran

Healthy Fats

- Avocados, guacamole, and avocado oil
- Fatty fish, including fresh or canned salmon, tuna, sardines, and lake trout

- Nuts, especially walnuts, peanuts, cashews, almonds, macadamia nuts, pecans, hazelnuts, and nut butters
- Oils, especially extra virgin olive oil (EVOO), safflower oil, grapeseed oil, sesame oil, and canola oil
- Olives
- Seeds, especially sunflower seeds, pumpkin seeds, ground flax seeds, chia seeds, hemp seeds, sesame seeds, and seed butters

Love Foods

- Ginger chews
- Ginger snaps
- Kombucha

Eating to Boost Bone Health

To maintain strong bones and help prevent osteopenia (thinning bones) and osteoporosis (thin bones that break easily), choose foods high in calcium, magnesium, vitamin D, potassium, vitamin C, zinc, and protein. Eating combination foods that contain two or more of these key nutrients can support bone health even more. Many of the foods listed here are super-bone foods, boasting a combination of several nutrients.

To maintain strong bones, include weight-bearing exercises in your MOVE plan, and choose these foods for strong bones.

Produce

- Bananas
- Broccoli
- Cabbage
- Calcium-fortified orange juice, grapefruit juice, or other juices

- Citrus fruits, including oranges, tangerines, and grapefruit
- Dark greens, including spinach, kale, arugula, bok choy, collards, dandelion greens, Swiss chard, and mustard greens (fresh or frozen)
- Figs
- Mushrooms
- Prunes
- Rhubarb

Proteins

- Beans and peas (legumes), including black beans, kidney beans, garbanzo beans, lentils, and others
- Calcium-fortified and vitamin D-fortified plant-based milks like soy milk, almond milk, pea milk, oat milk, and hemp milk
- Cheese
- Cottage cheese
- Eggs
- Fatty fish, including canned or fresh salmon, tuna, sardines, and lake trout
- Kefir
- Milk
- Nuts, especially walnuts, peanuts, cashews, almonds, macadamia nuts, pecans, hazelnuts, and nut butters
- Seeds, especially sunflower seeds, pumpkin seeds, ground flax seeds, chia seeds, hemp seeds, sesame seeds, and seed butters
- Soy-based foods including edamame, tofu, tempeh, miso, soy yogurt, and soy milk
- Yogurt

Grains and Starches

- Brown rice
- Corn tortillas
- English muffins
- Oats, including whole oat groats, steel-cut oats, oat bran, old-fashioned oats, and quick oats
- Quinoa
- Sweet potatoes, purple potatoes, and yams
- White and yellow potatoes
- Whole-wheat bread

Healthy Fats

- Avocados and guacamole
- Fatty fish, including canned or fresh salmon, tuna, sardines, and lake trout
- Nuts, especially walnuts, peanuts, cashews, almonds, macadamia nuts, pecans, hazelnuts, and nut butters
- Oils, especially extra virgin olive oil (EVOO), safflower oil, grapeseed oil, sesame oil, and canola oil
- Seeds, especially sunflower seeds, pumpkin seeds, ground flax seeds, chia seeds, hemp seeds, sesame seeds, and seed butters

Love Foods

- Dark chocolate, try a 1-ounce piece
- Low-fat frozen yogurt cups
- 100-calorie ice cream treats

Eating to Lower Inflammation

Chronic inflammation (slow, long-term inflammation lasting from months to years) is linked to many common diseases like heart disease, arthritis, diabetes, depression, and Alzheimer's disease. Choosing foods that may decrease inflammation in the body can boost your overall health and well-being.

The **2211** EAT plan is set up as an anti-inflammation plan because of its plant-based approach. Many plant-based compounds and anti-inflammatory fats help to lower inflammation in the body. Include these foods more frequently in the plan if you are looking to decrease inflammation.

Produce

- Beets
- Berries, including blueberries, blackberries, strawberries, raspberries, and others
- Broccoli
- Cabbage
- Cauliflower
- Cherries and tart cherry juice
- Citrus fruits, including oranges, tangerines, and grapefruit
- Grapes
- Greens-dark, leafy especially beet greens, Swiss chard, and cooked spinach
- Mushrooms
- Peppers
- Tomatoes

Proteins

- Beans and peas (legumes), including black beans, kidney beans, garbanzo beans, lentils, and others
- Eggs, especially omega-3 fortified eggs
- Fish, especially salmon, tuna, herring, sardines, trout, tilapia, shad, mullet, and pollock

- Hummus
- Nuts, especially walnuts, peanuts, cashews, almonds, macadamia nuts, pecans, hazelnuts, and nut butters
- Seeds, especially sunflower seeds, pumpkin seeds, ground flax seeds, chia seeds, hemp seeds, sesame seeds, and seed butters

Grains and Starches

- Sweet potatoes, purple potatoes, and yams
- White, yellow, and purple potatoes
- Whole-grain bread like whole wheat, rye, or oat
- Whole-grain cereal like wheat flakes, toasted oats, or rye flakes

Healthy Fats

- Avocados
- Fish, especially salmon, tuna, herring, sardines, trout, tilapia, shad, mullet, and pollock
- Nuts, especially walnuts, peanuts, cashews, almonds, macadamia nuts, pecans, hazelnuts, and nut butters
- Oils, especially extra virgin olive oil (EVOO), safflower oil, grapeseed oil, sesame oil, and canola oil
- Seeds, especially sunflower seeds, pumpkin seeds, ground flax seeds, chia seeds, hemp seeds, sesame seeds, and seed butters

Love Foods

- Dark chocolate, try a 1-ounce piece

Top 22 Foods to Put in Your Grocery Cart

Many foods come up again and again in this chapter as beneficial foods to help manage health conditions and optimize well-being. Which foods do I recommend you eat more often? Here's my starter list of 22 health-enhancing and budget-friendly foods to add to your grocery cart. This is not an exclusive list, but if you haven't added some of these foods to your grocery list, give them a try.

Produce

- Berries, such as blackberries, blueberries, raspberries, and strawberries
- Broccoli
- Carrots
- Onions
- Oranges, grapefruit, and other citrus fruits and juices
- Spinach, kale, and other dark greens
- Tomatoes and tomato products like pasta sauce and salsa

Protein

- Beans, including black beans, lentils, and chickpeas
- Eggs
- Fish, especially canned or fresh salmon, tuna, and sardines
- Lean meats like chicken breast, turkey breast, pork loin, and beef sirloin
- Milk and plant-based milks
- Nuts, seeds, and nut and seed butters
- Soy foods including edamame, tofu, and tempeh
- Yogurt and plant-based yogurts

Grains and Starches

- Corn and whole corn foods like corn tortillas
- Potatoes, sweet potatoes, purple potatoes, and yams
- Rice, especially brown rice
- Whole-grain breads, cereals, and crackers
- Whole grains like oats, barley, and quinoa

Healthy Fats

- Avocados
- Healthy oils like olive oil (and olives), avocado oil, canola oil, and peanut oil and oil-based salad dressings

Next up, you'll learn how to plan meals and put together simple, fast, low-cost, easy meals. You'll be surprised by how simple it is to build a 2211 meal using foods you may already have in your pantry, refrigerator, and freezer. Let's get started.

5

Meal Planning Made Easy

N ow that you've taken inventory of your food options, it's time to plan for fast, simple, easy-to-make meals that fit the 2211 plan. This is where the 2-minute miracle comes in. Here's how it works.

Each evening when you're relaxing, in the kitchen, or watching your favorite show, take two minutes to think about tomorrow. It's amazing how just two minutes of your time and attention can change how a whole day plays out. For the EAT part of your tomorrow, jot down the following:

- 6 cups of produce I can eat tomorrow
- 3 protein options I can eat tomorrow
- 3 grains (especially whole grains) I can eat tomorrow
- 3 healthy fats I can eat tomorrow

Next, consider meals you could make (or combine foods together to make fast meals) to get your meal bases covered.

By that, I mean you set up the framework for your meals for the next day. Here's an example from my kitchen:

- Produce options: orange juice, bananas, broccoli, salad greens, apples
- Protein options: eggs, Greek yogurt, tofu, chicken breast, shredded cheddar cheese, shredded Parmesan cheese, milk, slivered almonds, peanuts
- Grains: whole-grain bread, whole-wheat crackers, potatoes, whole-grain pasta, popcorn
- Healthy fats: Italian dressing, olive oil, avocados

Then, frame your **2211** meals on these foods. For example, from the foods just mentioned, I can make a simple plan for tomorrow's meals. Add your own love foods when you like.

Breakfast

1 cup orange juice + 1 banana + 2 boiled eggs + 1 slice whole-grain toast + 2 cups of coffee with milk

The **2211** breakdown:

2 produce: 1 cup orange juice + 1 banana

2 protein: 2 boiled eggs (2 ounces protein) + 1 cup milk with my coffee (1 ounce protein)

1 grain: 1 slice whole grain toast

1 healthy fat: eggs contain a healthy fat serving

Lunch

2 cups salad + ¼ cup slivered almonds + ¼ cup shredded cheddar cheese + 1 Tablespoon Italian dressing + ½ cup whole-grain crackers

The 2211 breakdown:

2 produce: 2 cups salad

2 protein: ¼ cup slivered almonds + ¼ cup shredded cheddar cheese (2 ounces protein + 1 healthy fat)

1 grain: 10 whole-grain crackers

1 healthy fat: 1 Tablespoon Italian dressing

Love: 1 ounce chocolate

Dinner

3 ounces chicken breast + 2 cups steamed broccoli + ½ cup whole- grain pasta with olive oil and a pinch of shredded Parmesan cheese

The 2211 breakdown:

2 produce: 2 cups steamed broccoli

2+ protein: 3 ounces grilled chicken breast

1 grain: ½ cup cooked pasta

1 healthy fat: 1 teaspoon olive oil

Love: 5 ounces red wine

Bev's Food Options

Let's look at another example of simple meal planning from my client Bev. Here is a one-day plan using her favorite foods:

- Produce: salad mix, grape tomatoes, bananas, oranges, fresh broccoli, fresh cauliflower, canned pears, applesauce, frozen blueberries, and frozen green beans
- Proteins: ground turkey, frozen veggie burgers, soy milk, Greek yogurt, mozzarella cheese sticks, and peanut butter

- Grains: whole-grain hamburger buns, pretzels, corn tortillas, snack pack microwave popcorn packs, canned corn, and granola
- Healthy Fats: peanut butter, Italian dressing, avocados, and olive oil

Here is her day's menu:

Breakfast

Yogurt parfait with 2/3 cup Greek yogurt, 1 cup blueberries, 1 sliced banana, and ¼ cup granola with nuts

The **2211** breakdown:

> 2 produce: 1 cup blueberries + 1 banana
>
> 2 protein: 2/3 cup Greek yogurt (2 ounces protein)
>
> 1 grain: ¼ cup granola
>
> 1 healthy fat: nuts in the granola

Lunch

1 soft taco with cooked ground turkey and avocado, 1 cup chopped cauliflower, and 1 cup canned pears

The **2211** breakdown:

> 2 produce: 1 cup chopped cauliflower + 1 cup canned pears
>
> 2 protein: ½ cup ground turkey (2 ounces protein)
>
> 1 grain: 1 corn tortilla
>
> 1 healthy fat: 1/2 sliced avocado

Snack: 1 sliced apple + 1 cheese stick

The 2211 breakdown:

   1 produce: 1 sliced apple

   1 protein: 1 cheese stick (1 ounce protein)

Dinner

1 veggie burger with a whole-grain bun + 1 cup salad/tomatoes + 1 Tablespoon oil and vinegar dressing + 1 sliced orange

The 2211 breakdown:

   2 produce: 1 cup salad + 1 orange

   2 protein: 1 veggie burger patty (2 ounces protein)

   1 grain: 1 whole-grain bun

   1 healthy fat: 1 Tablespoon oil and vinegar dressing

   Love: 1 snack-size ice cream cup

Now it's your turn.

1. Download the 2-minute miracle weekly planning sheet from *eatmovegroove.com*.

2. Complete the checklist for tomorrow's EAT plan. Keep this sheet handy for the remainder of the week.

3. You're ready to go.

You can see that eating well on the 2211 plan doesn't have to take a lot of time or energy. Making a healthy 2211 meal can be as simple as combining foods you have on hand.

Start with Your Pantry, Fridge, and Freezer

A super simple way to build a 2211 meal is to look no further than your pantry or freezer. When you're in a rush or just don't feel like cooking, you can easily turn the ingredients you already have on hand into **2211** meals. Some of these foods, like frozen meals, soups, stews, or other mixed foods, are also high in protein. Look for choices that contain at least 2 ounces of protein, or 15 grams of protein on a food label.

Sometimes eating frozen meals or canned soups or stews as part of your **2211** plan can save time, money, and energy—three precious commodities in life. Here are a few single-serving frozen meals and soups that provide at least 2 ounces of protein. Start with your frozen, canned, or packaged meal. Then add a few additional foods to meet your **2211** plan, and you're all set.

Be mindful that many processed meals and soups may contain higher amounts of salt. Remedy this by adding more produce to the meal (especially fresh or frozen fruits and vegetables). You'll also be upping the fiber content of the meal by boosting the produce.

Fast and Easy 2211 Meals from the Freezer or Pantry

Progresso Lentil & Roasted Vegetable Soup: 14 grams of protein for the can

Add-ins for your 2211 meal: 1 slice toasted whole-grain bread, 1 cup grapes, and 1 teaspoon olive oil–based spread

The **2211** breakdown:

    2 produce: 1 cup vegetables in the soup + 1 cup grapes

    2+ protein: 2 ounces protein in the soup + 1 ounce cheese (3 ounces protein)

    1 whole grain: 1 slice whole-grain bread

    1 healthy fat: 1 teaspoon olive oil–based spread on bread

Chef's Cupboard Chunky Grilled Chicken & Sausage Gumbo Soup: 14 grams of protein for the can

Add-ins for your 2211 meal: 1 cup baby carrots, 1 apple, and a handful of peanuts

The **2211** breakdown:

- 2 produce: 1 cup baby carrots + 1 apple
- 2 protein: protein in the soup + peanuts (3 ounces protein)
- 1 grain: rice in the soup
- 1 healthy fat: peanuts

Lean Cuisine Tortilla Crusted Fish: 15 grams of protein

Add-ins for your 2211 meal: 1 sliced mango, 1 cup cauliflower, and 5 olives

The **2211** breakdown:

- 2 produce: 1 sliced mango + 1 cup cauliflower
- 2 protein: fish in the meal (2 ounces protein)
- 1 grain: rice/corn mix in the meal
- 1 healthy fat: 5 olives

Michelina's Chicken Fajita Bowl: 17 grams of protein

Add-ins for your 2211 meal: 1 orange and 1/2 avocado

The **2211** breakdown:

- 2 produce: veggies in the meal + 1 orange
- 2 protein: chicken in the meal (2+ ounces protein)
- 1 grain: rice in the meal
- 1 healthy fat: 1/2 avocado

Amy's Bowls, Chili Mac: 15 grams of protein

Add-ins for your 2211 meal: 1 pear and a handful of almonds

The **2211** breakdown:

- 2 produce: tomatoes in the meal + 1 pear
- 2 protein: protein in the meal (2 ounces) + almonds (1 ounce)
- 1 grain: pasta in the meal
- 1 healthy fat: almonds

Banquet Spaghetti and Meatballs: 16 grams of protein

Add-ins for your 2211 meal: 2 cups mixed salad greens, 1 Tablespoon Italian dressing

The **2211** breakdown:

- 2 produce: 2 cups salad greens
- 2 protein: protein in the meal (2+ ounces protein)
- 1 grain: pasta in the meal
- 1 healthy fat: 1 Tablespoon Italian dressing

Whole & Simple Southwestern Style Chicken Quinoa Bowl: 16 grams of protein

Add-ins for your 2211 meal: 1 ½ cups steamed mixed veggies, 1 Tablespoon ground flax seeds

The **2211** breakdown:

- 2 produce: ½ cup veggies in the meal + 1 ½ cup steamed mixed veggies
- 2 protein: protein in the meal (2+ ounces protein)
- 1 grain: quinoa in the meal
- 1 healthy fat: add 1 Tablespoon ground flax seeds to the bowl

Healthy Choice Simply Steamers Chicken Tikka Masala: 17 grams of protein

Add-ins for your 2211 meal: 1 cup melon, ½ whole-grain pita, handful of cashews

The **2211** breakdown:

- 2 produce: veggies in the meal + 1 cup melon
- 2 protein: protein in the meal + cashews (3 ounces protein)
- 1 grain: ½ pita
- 1 healthy fat: cashews

Stouffer's Chicken and Broccoli Pasta Bake: 19 grams of protein

Add-ins for your 2211 meal: 2 cups spinach salad and 1 Tablespoon raspberry vinaigrette

The **2211** breakdown:

- 2 produce: 2 cups spinach salad
- 2 protein: chicken in the meal (2+ ounces protein)
- 1 grain: pasta in the meal
- 1 healthy fat: 1 Tablespoon raspberry vinaigrette

Considering canned soups or frozen meals gets back to your how with the **2211** plan. How do you like to eat? You may be a cook and prefer to cook your own meals. Or maybe you don't enjoy cooking or don't have much time to spend in the kitchen and prefer to boost frozen meals or partially prepared meals to hit the **2211** targets. Either way, you can utilize the simple ideas of the **2211** plan, just as you see with the frozen meals and prepared soups and stews just listed.

In the next chapter, you'll find a one-week meal plan to get you going on the 2211 plan: a week's grocery list, ideas for prepping some foods ahead to save time, and easy, fast recipes using common foods and ingredients to accompany the menu plans. Let's get eating with 2211.

6

Eating on the Go

L ife can be hectic and sometimes unpredictable. Our changing schedules often dictate when, where, and what we
eat, which foods are available to us, and how the food is
prepared. Even so, we can plan for these times. When time
is crunched and we find ourselves tired and hungry at work,
on the road, at convenience stores, driving through fast-food
stops, eating at restaurants, and even on road trips, we can still
eat well. Once again, as little as two minutes of preparation
can pay off in a big way.

Pack Meals and Snacks

If you're away from home for lunch or any other meal, you
can put together fast and easy cooler meals that will satisfy
you and save you money too. Pack them the night before so
all you have to do in the morning is grab your cooler bag and
be on your way.

You'll also save money. On average, making your own lunch
usually costs less than $5—you'll often pay at least twice that

amount if you eat out for lunch. That adds up to a huge savings. Eating the **2211** way means you're building your wealth and your health at the same time.

Simple Sandwich and Wrap Meals

A sandwich or a wrap is a fast and simple way to put together an on-the-go meal. Add a piece of fruit, a vegetable, and a love food if you want and you have an easy, no-nonsense meal. It's the meal I often pack for lunch when I know I've got a busy day.

Here are some quick options, all under $5 per meal:

PB&J Meal

Peanut butter and jelly sandwich on whole-wheat bread

1 cup baby carrots

1 cup grapes

Turkey, Cheese, and Pesto Wrap Meal

Turkey, cheese, and pesto wrap (see recipe in this book)

1 cup sliced sweet peppers

1 apple

Hummus Pita Pocket Meal

Hummus pita pocket

1 cup sliced cucumbers

1 peach

Chicken Pita Meal

Half a whole-wheat pita with grilled chicken and romaine lettuce

Ranch dressing

1 cup sliced cucumbers

1 orange

Tuna Salad Meal

Tuna salad sandwich on whole wheat with lettuce

1 cup sliced carrots and celery

1 cup cherries

Other Fast Lunch Options

You can make so many easy, inexpensive options for fast meals. You might heat up leftovers or a frozen meal in the microwave at work or pack a hearty salad in a thermal bag. By planning ahead, you can eat well, save money, and decrease food waste at the same time.

- Pack leftovers. Don't leave your dinner leftovers languishing in the fridge. Bring them along for lunch. Add a piece of fruit or some sliced veggies to round out the meal.

- Grab a healthy frozen meal and heat it up in the microwave for a fast lunch. Add a piece of fruit for something sweet.

- Bring a bowl of hearty soup along with some whole-grain crackers and fruit.

- Build a healthy bowl with a grain or starch (rice, quinoa, or sweet potatoes), add veggies, and top it with a protein source like chicken, pork loin, eggs, or tofu. Finish it off with a drizzle of olive oil, sliced avocados, or chopped nuts to add healthy fat.

A few other options to consider—

Burrito Meal

    Frozen bean and rice burrito

    1 cup chopped broccoli

    1 apple

Soup On-the-Go Meal

    1 single-serving container vegetable beef barley soup

    1 cheese stick

    1 cup grapes

Salmon and Sides Meal

    1 single-serving salmon pack

    1 cup salad mix with vinaigrette

    10 whole-grain crackers

    2 clementines

Simple Salad Meal

    2 cups Simple Salad (see recipe in this book)

    1 slice whole-grain bread

Super Salad in a Jar Meal (see recipe in this book)

    1 banana

Convenience Store Meals

Sometimes all you can manage for lunch or another meal is a quick stop at a convenience store. You can still eat a healthy meal. You'll find plenty of options that work with the 2211 plan. Just keep produce and protein top of mind.

Convenience store tips—

- Look for produce wherever you can find it, including fresh fruit, snack pack veggies, canned fruit cups, dried fruit packs, and 100% juices.

- Add on proteins, such as single-serving packs of nuts, sunflower seeds, hummus, jerky, boiled eggs, cheese sticks, cheese and cracker packs, dried soybeans, yogurt cups, and protein bars.

- Check out easy-to-eat meals like prepared salads, sub sandwiches, bean and cheese burritos, chicken or beef tacos and burritos, grilled chicken sandwiches, and turkey, ham and cheese, roast beef, and tuna or egg salad sandwiches.

11 Convenience Store Meal Ideas

- Hummus and crackers pack
  Banana
  Baby carrots

- Grilled chicken sandwich
  Fruit/vegetable juice (choose 100% juice)

- Single-serving package of nuts
  Cheese stick
  Whole-grain crackers
  Orange

- Bean and cheese burrito
  Apple

- Sub sandwich
  100% cranapple juice

- Single-serving sushi
  Single-serving nuts
  Baby carrots

- Premade salad with eggs, cheese, and turkey
  Banana

- Vegetable soup
  Crackers
  Cheese stick
  Orange

- Slice of pizza
  Sliced veggie cup
  Banana

- Chicken burrito
  Side salad
  Apple

- Roast beef and cheese or tuna sandwich on whole-grain bread
  Baby carrots
  Banana

Fast-Food Fueling

Zipping through a drive-through is sometimes the fastest and easiest way to grab a meal on the go, especially when you're traveling.

You may not always have a lot of options, but whenever possible, avoid fried foods and sugary drinks. Instead, go for sub sandwiches, pitas, grilled sandwiches, salads, single burgers, tacos, or veggie and bean burritos. Look for fruit and veggie sides like apple slices, baby carrots, baked potatoes and side salads. For a beverage, try coffee, iced tea, sugar-free sodas, milk, or 100 percent juices. If you want something sweet, try fruit and yogurt parfaits and smoothies made with real fruit.

Consider ordering the smaller or kid's version of meals when eating fast-food. Even if you eat the french fries, the total amount you consume will be less. For example, a typical fast-food double burger with medium fries and a medium drink can average around 1,200 calories. But if you choose a regular hamburger, small fries, apple slices, and a small 1 percent milk, the total comes to under 500 calories. At the same time, you're getting one serving of produce and 3 ounces of protein. That's a simple swap. Being aware of portion sizes makes a big difference in your overall health and well-being over time.

11 Fast-Food Meal Ideas on the Go

- Grilled hamburger, turkey burger, or veggie burger
  Side salad with vinaigrette dressing
  100% fruit juice

- Grilled chicken salad with vinaigrette dressing
  Apple slices

- Bean, chicken, or beef burrito
  100% fruit juice

- Grilled chicken pieces
  Cole slaw
  Green beans
  Baked beans

- Kid's/junior hamburger or cheeseburger meal
  Small fries
  Side of apples or applesauce

- Salad bowl with black beans, rice, guacamole, and salsa
  Iced tea

- Turkey and veggie sub sandwich
  Side of baked chips

- Salad with ham, cheese, veggies, and vinaigrette dressing
  100% fruit juice

- Grilled chicken sandwich
  Side of fresh fruit or applesauce

- Roast beef sandwich
  100 % fruit juice

- Egg and cheese wrap
  100% fruit juice

Restaurant Meals

When dining at sit-down restaurants, you can easily find lots of options to meet your produce and protein first lifestyle. Ask your server about options for side dishes that may not be on the menu. You may find you can order fresh fruit, steamed vegetables, or side salads instead of sides like french fries. Even if a menu item comes fried, you may be able to ask for it to be grilled, a much healthier option.

Being proactive and advocating for your health and well-being when you eat out can be a game-changer for you. And remember, occasionally you may be celebrating special events, enjoying birthday meals, or just having a relaxing dinner. Eating meals you enjoy, even if they don't fit into the 2211 lifestyle, is important too.

11 Sit-Down Meal Ideas

- Grilled chicken breast
  Steamed vegetables
  Baked potato
  Side salad with vinaigrette dressing

- Grilled salmon, tuna, or shrimp
  Steamed broccoli
  Rice
  Orange juice

- Beans and rice with salsa
  Side salad with light dressing
  Side of fresh fruit

- Shrimp and veggie skewers
  Rice
  Side salad with light dressing

- Veggie-based soup such as minestrone, tomato, or
  vegetable beef
  Side salad with light dressing
  Whole-grain roll

- Petite sirloin steak or pork loin
  Steamed mixed veggies
  Corn
  Side salad with light dressing

- Spaghetti and meatballs
  Steamed mixed veggies
  Side salad with vinaigrette

- Fajitas with tofu, beef, chicken, or fish
  Black beans
  Rice

- Grilled fish tacos with salsa
  Side salad with light dressing
  Pineapple juice

- Tofu and vegetable stir-fry
  Brown rice

- Hummus plate with sliced veggies, olives, yogurt, and pita bread

Road Trip Fueling

Headed off on a road trip? Just as you pack your clothes, make it a habit to pack a cooler and food box for the car. The goal is to have plenty of healthy options when you're on the road. This will not only boost your health, but it will also save you time, money, and the hassle of finding healthy food at every stop. Even if you mix and match your meals—eating some meals from your car and eating out for others—the small amount of time it takes to set up your food in advance pays off fast.

An extra benefit of bringing your own food when you travel is that it gives you the opportunity to stop anywhere when you're ready for a break. Pull over at a rest area or find a spot near a lake or in a park where you can MOVE as well as EAT. This way, you control not only when and what you eat but also how you MOVE your body. At a minimum, take a walk to get yourself moving. If you're with family or friends, bring along a soccer ball, football, frisbee, or hacky sack and get some exercise while you take a meal break. It's fun and great for your body.

Here's what to pack along in the car, on a bus, on a train, or in an airplane.

Travel Cooler

- Single-serving 100% fruit and veggie juices
- Precut carrots, peppers, cherry tomatoes, cucumbers, celery, cauliflower, and other veggies
- Grapes, apples, oranges, cherries, bananas, and other fruit
- Yogurt cups and squeezable yogurts
- Drinkable kefir and yogurt drinks
- Cheese sticks and slices
- Hummus
- Edamame
- Guacamole packs
- Ham, turkey, or roast beef and cheese tortilla roll-ups
- Premade sandwiches

Travel Food Box

- Nuts
- Nut butters
- Pumpkin seeds and sunflower seeds
- Trail mix
- Jerky (meat or veggie)
- Granola bars
- Protein bars
- Fruit bars and 100% fruit rolls
- Tortilla chips
- Popcorn
- Dried fruit
- Whole-grain crackers
- Fig bars

No matter where you are off to, or how you're getting there, with a little planning, you can either bring your **2211** meals with you or find options that work for you on the road. That's the simplicity of the **2211** EAT plan and lifestyle. It gives you the peace of mind to know you're taking care of yourself every day in simple ways.

7

One-Week Meal Plan and Recipes

I n this chapter, you'll find a one-week meal plan with a grocery list and easy-to-make recipes. These foods taste great, use common ingredients you can easily find, and are fast to make. The recipes are delicious and accessible, so you can use the one-week plan as a way to put 2211 into practice.

These meal plans help you get into the rhythm of the 2211 lifestyle. You can modify them to add your own favorite foods, your own flair, and your own spices, flavors, and combinations you enjoy. If you prefer to choose all plant-based options, for example, you can easily make that switch. You may prefer plant-based cheeses or choose baked tofu instead of turkey breast. You may prefer to eat more apples or oranges if you already have a refrigerator full of these fruits. That's fine. The meal plans and recipes are flexible. I encourage you to modify them to meet your own preferences.

This simple one-week meal plan and the recipes are your foundation for launching the 2211 EAT plan. You'll find more meal planning ideas, recipes, and EAT ideas online at *eatmovegroove.com.*

Your Grocery List

Shopping with a grocery list in hand is one simple tool that makes it easier to enjoy the 2211 lifestyle. Spending a little time planning ahead often means you come home with plenty of fruits, vegetables, whole grains, and high-quality proteins to build your 2211 meals.

Step 1: Make your grocery list. If you usually grocery shop at the same store (or online), shop in the order you move around the store. For example, if you shop in the produce area first (I recommend this), start there and move your way around the store as you typically do. That's how you'll make your grocery list too.

Step 2: Check off items you already have in your kitchen, including staples, spices, and seasonings.

Step 3: Let's go shopping. This list will provide you with all the foods needed in the one-week meal plan for a family of four. Modify the list based on your preferences—do what works best for you. Purchase fresh, canned, frozen, and dried options that meet your budget and your likes.

One-Week Meal Plan Grocery List

Fresh Fruits and Vegetables

Fruits

- Apples
- Avocados
- Bananas

- Blueberries (and any berries you enjoy)
- Clementines
- Grapes
- Lemons
- Melon (any you enjoy)
- Oranges
- Peaches (or canned in juice or light syrup)
- Pears (or canned in juice or light syrup)
- Pineapple (or canned in juice or light syrup)
- Strawberries

Vegetables

- Asparagus
- Basil (fresh or dried)
- Broccoli (fresh or frozen)
- Carrots
- Celery
- Cherry or grape tomatoes
- Cucumbers
- Dark salad greens (romaine, kale, arugula, others)
- Ginger (fresh or dried)
- Green onions
- Mushrooms (fresh or canned)
- Onions (fresh or frozen)
- Potatoes (fresh or frozen diced potatoes)
- Spinach (fresh or frozen)
- Summer squash
- Sweet peppers (fresh or frozen)
- Sweet potatoes

Refrigerated Foods

- Chicken breasts or thighs (fresh, precooked, or frozen)
- Cheese: shredded cheddar, feta, mozzarella (shredded or sticks), cheddar slices, and pepper jack block
- Cottage cheese, low-fat
- Eggs
- Hummus
- Milk or plant-based milk
- Orange juice, calcium-fortified
- Salmon filets (fresh or frozen)
- Tilapia or other whitefish you enjoy (fresh or frozen)
- Tofu, extra-firm
- Turkey breast, sliced
- Turkey, chicken, pork, or veggie Italian sausage (fresh or frozen)
- Yogurt, Greek-style or plant-based

Frozen Foods

- Blueberries
- Burgers (beef, turkey, or veggie)
- Edamame, shelled
- Mixed vegetables
- Peaches
- Pizza, small thin crust or pizza crust
- Spinach

Pantry Items

- Bagels, whole-grain
- Bread, whole-grain
- Brown or white rice
- Buns, whole-grain

- Chickpeas, canned
- Crackers, whole-grain
- English muffins, whole-grain
- Fruit, canned (peaches, pears, pineapple, or any you enjoy)
- Granola bars, fruit bars, nut bars
- Granola cereal
- Great northern beans, canned
- Lentils, dry
- Nuts (walnuts, slivered almonds, and any other nuts you enjoy)
- Oatmeal
- Olives, diced
- Pasta sauce
- Peanut butter (creamy) and any nut butters you enjoy
- Pesto
- Picante sauce (or salsa)
- Pita bread, whole-wheat
- Seeds (chia, sunflower, and any other seeds you enjoy)
- Spaghetti or pasta, whole-wheat
- Tomatoes, diced canned
- Tortilla chips
- Vegetable juice
- Vegetable stock
- Vinaigrette dressing and other light salad dressings you enjoy

Check Your Kitchen for These Staples

Spices

- Bay leaves
- Chili powder
- Cinnamon

- Cumin
- Garlic cloves, minced garlic, or garlic powder
- Garlic salt
- Ginger (fresh or dried)
- Pepper
- Pizza seasoning
- Salt
- Spice mixes you enjoy (African, Greek, Indian, Italian)

Other Staples

- Brown sugar
- Honey
- Maple syrup
- Mustard, Dijon
- Oils: avocado, olive, canola
- Red chili sauce, spicy sweet
- Soy sauce, light
- Vinegar: balsamic, red wine, rice

One-Week Meal Plan

*The asterisk * means the recipe for this dish is found later in this book.*

Monday

> **Breakfast:** Blueberry and Cinnamon Overnight Oats* and orange juice
>
> **Lunch:** Simple Salad* with whole-grain crackers
>
> **Dinner:** Citrus Salmon* with broccoli, brown rice, and sliced oranges

Tuesday

Breakfast: Garden Scramble* with whole-grain toast

Lunch: Brown Rice, Chickpea, and Veggie Bowl* with grapes

Dinner: Slow Cooker Chicken Chili* with corn tortilla chips, pineapple, and carrot sticks

Wednesday

Breakfast: Morning Breeze Smoothie* with a fruit and nut granola bar

Lunch: Super Salad in a Jar* with Basic Balsamic Vinaigrette*

Dinner: Fast Fried Rice*

Thursday

Breakfast: Egg and Cheese Wrap* with avocado slices, vegetable juice, and strawberries

Lunch: Turkey, Cheese, and Pesto Roll* with pepper slices and apple

Dinner: Veg Out Pizza* with sliced pears

Friday

Breakfast: Sunshine Breakfast Bowl*

Lunch: Hummus Pocket* with sliced cucumbers and peach

Dinner: Tilapia with Tomato-Basil Salsa and Roasted Potatoes* with a side salad

Saturday

Breakfast: Blender Banana Milk* with a whole-grain bagel with peanut butter and 2 clementines

Lunch: Slow Cooker Lentil and Veggie Soup* with a side salad and pita bread

Dinner: Grilled burgers on buns with Cinnamon Fruit Salad* and grilled asparagus

Sunday

Breakfast: Veggie and Egg Muffin Cups* with a whole-grain English muffin and banana

Lunch: Tofu, Broccoli, and Sweet Potato Bowl* with Peanut Sauce* and melon slices

Dinner: Slow Cooker Sausage and Veggie Pasta*

RECIPES

Breakfasts

Blueberry and Cinnamon Overnight Oats

Makes 2 servings

I love making overnight oats for the next morning at the same time I'm preparing dinner. Try mixed berries or canned or frozen peaches. You might enjoy flavored yogurt or add a teaspoon of honey or maple syrup to plain yogurt for a burst of sweetness.

INGREDIENTS:

½	cup dry oats
2	teaspoons chia seeds
1	teaspoon cinnamon
1½	cups plain or flavored Greek yogurt
2	cups frozen blueberries

DIRECTIONS:

1. In 2 16-ounce jars, add half of each ingredient in the order listed.
2. Refrigerate overnight.
3. Enjoy cold or warm up for 45 to 60 seconds in the microwave.

2211 MEAL PLAN SERVINGS

Add 1 cup orange juice to make a meal

2	1 cup blueberries + 1 cup orange juice
2	⅔ cup Greek yogurt
1	¼ cup dry oats
1	1 teaspoon chia seeds

Garden Scramble

Makes 2 servings

Take inventory of your refrigerator and make this recipe as a way to use up produce that's been hanging around. I start with dark greens and chop up leftover broccoli, tomatoes, mushrooms, or any other veggies I have. This is a way to clean out the fridge and decrease food waste with a great-tasting breakfast.

INGREDIENTS:

3	cups chopped fresh spinach or dark greens or 1 cup frozen or cooked greens
1	cup chopped peppers (or any veggies you have)
2	Tablespoons chopped onions
4	eggs
½	cup milk
¼	cup shredded cheddar cheese
2	teaspoons avocado, olive, or canola oil

DIRECTIONS:

1. In a small bowl, crack the eggs, add milk, and mix well. Set aside.
2. In a skillet, heat oil on medium until hot (about 1 minute).
3. Add peppers and onions and sauté for 2 to 3 minutes, or until soft.
4. Add spinach or greens and sauté for another 1 to 2 minutes, or until cooked down.
5. Add egg mixture, stirring frequently for 2 to 3 minutes, or until eggs are cooked through.
6. Top with shredded cheddar cheese.

2211 MEAL PLAN SERVINGS

Add 1 slice whole-grain toast to make a meal

2	2 cups spinach/peppers/onions
2	2 eggs + milk
1	1 slice whole-grain toast
1	oil and eggs

Morning Breeze Smoothie

Makes 2 servings

This smoothie is quick and easy to make and tastes so refreshing. Make it at home in your blender for a fraction of the price you'd pay ordering it out. Use any frozen fruit and 100% juice you have on hand. Look for calcium-fortified juice when possible. No yogurt? Try your favorite milk or kefir instead. Grab a granola bar with this smoothie and you're out the door in just a couple of minutes. For a quick snack, I often cut the portions to ½ cup each of fruit, juice, and milk, and whip up a refreshing afternoon treat.

INGREDIENTS:

2	cups frozen peaches
2	cups 100% orange juice
2	cups Greek yogurt (plain, vanilla, or fruit)

DIRECTIONS:

1. Pour all ingredients into a blender.
2. Blend well on high until smooth.

2211 MEAL PLAN SERVINGS

Add 1 granola bar with nuts and seeds to make a meal

2	1 cup peaches + 1 cup orange juice
2	1 cup yogurt
1	1 granola bar
1	nuts/seeds in granola bar

Fast Egg and Cheese Wrap

Makes 2 servings

These wraps are a fast, filling breakfast starter. Microwaving eggs saves time in the morning. You can even add a microwavable sausage link or veggie patty.

INGREDIENTS:

2	eggs
2	slices cheddar cheese or your favorite cheese
2	small or "street" corn or flour tortillas
1	avocado, sliced
	salsa

DIRECTIONS:

1. In a small glass bowl, scramble the eggs.
2. Cover and microwave for 1 minute.
3. Check for doneness and cook for up to 60 more seconds until the eggs are no longer runny.
4. Place the tortillas on plates and top each with 1 slice of cheese. Add half the scrambled eggs to each tortilla.
5. Microwave for 30 seconds to melt the cheese.
6. Top with half the sliced avocado and salsa to taste.

2211 MEAL PLAN SERVINGS

Add 1 cup vegetable juice and 1 cup strawberries to make a meal

2	1 cup vegetable juice + 1 cup strawberries
2	1 egg + 1 slice cheese
1	1 tortilla
1	sliced avocado/egg

Sunshine Breakfast Bowl

Makes 2 servings

This bowl is one of my favorite breakfasts. It's so simple, delicious, and a perfect mix of **2211** servings. Plus, there's nothing to cook! Try it with berries and bananas or use any fresh, canned, or frozen fruit you have on hand.

INGREDIENTS:

1½	cups Greek yogurt
2	cups fresh or frozen berries
2	bananas, sliced
½	cup granola
4	Tablespoons walnuts or other nuts
½	teaspoon cinnamon

DIRECTIONS:

1. In two medium bowls, add half the berries on one side and half the sliced bananas on the other.
2. Top each bowl with ¾ cup yogurt.
3. Sprinkle ¼ cup granola, 2 Tablespoons walnuts, and ¼ teaspoon cinnamon on top of each bowl.

2211 MEAL PLAN SERVINGS

2	1 cup berries and 1 banana
2	¾ cup Greek yogurt
1	¼ cup granola
1	2 Tablespoons walnuts

Veggie Egg Muffin Cups

Makes 6 servings (2 muffin cups per serving)

Here's another opportunity to use up produce in your fridge or clean out the freezer and serve a larger group. If you like, add sausage, bacon, chopped ham, or seasoned veggie crumbles. Top with salsa, hot sauce, or your favorite sauces. After the egg muffin cups cool, you can freeze for up to two months. Just place them in the fridge the night before you eat them, and microwave for 1 minute.

INGREDIENTS:

8	eggs
½	cup milk
½	cup shredded cheese of your choice
4	cups fresh spinach or other greens (or 1 cup frozen greens)
½	cup chopped onions
2	cups chopped mushrooms, peppers, or other veggies (whatever is in your fridge)
2	teaspoons avocado oil, olive, or canola oil
	Salt and pepper

DIRECTIONS:

1. Preheat the oven to 350 degrees.
2. In a large bowl, mix eggs and milk until blended. Set aside.
3. In a large skillet, heat oil over medium for 1 minute, or until hot.
4. Add onions and cook for 2 to 3 minutes, stirring frequently.
5. Add greens and veggies and sauté for 2 to 3 minutes, or until soft.

6. Spray 12 muffin tins with cooking spray or use a nonstick muffin tin.
7. Divide cooked vegetables evenly in the bottom of muffin tins.
8. Pour egg mixture evenly over vegetables and top with shredded cheese.
9. Bake for 15 to 20 minutes, or until eggs are set and begin to brown.
10. Salt and pepper to taste.

2211 MEAL PLAN SERVINGS

Add a whole-grain English muffin and a banana to make a meal

2	1 cup veggies in the egg cups + 1 banana
2	2 egg cups
1	1 whole-grain English muffin
1	oil/eggs

Easy Blender Banana Milk

Makes 2 servings

If you haven't tried banana milk, here's your chance to give it a whirl. When I first made it, I was surprised at how fabulous it tasted. It's a simple way to mix produce and protein for breakfast, or for a midafternoon snack. This is a refreshing snack after exercise too. Drink after preparing so the bananas stay fresh. For a single serving, simply cut the ingredients in half.

INGREDIENTS:

2	cups milk of choice
2	medium bananas (soft, but not brown)
2	teaspoons vanilla extract
2	teaspoons honey
	Handful of ice cubes

DIRECTIONS:

1. Place all ingredients in a blender.
2. Blend on high until smooth. Strain if desired.
3. Pour into two glasses.

2211 MEAL PLAN SERVINGS

Add ½ whole-grain bagel with 2 Tablespoons nut butter and 2 clementines to make a meal

2	1 banana + 2 clementines
2	1 cup milk + 2 Tablespoons nut butter
1	½ whole grain bagel
1	nut butter

Lunches

Simple Salad

Makes 2 servings

How many times have you thought that a salad you eat in a restaurant tastes so much better than homemade salads? Me too—but not with this Simple Salad! Add any greens and veggies you like (or try a packaged salad mix), then add in edamame and nuts or seeds. Top with homemade vinaigrette dressing (see recipe in this section). Enjoy with whole-grain bread or crackers.

INGREDIENTS:

2	cups dark greens (spinach, romaine, kale, or any dark greens)
2	cups chopped veggies (carrots, cucumbers, peppers, broccoli, and any veggies)
1	cup edamame, shelled
½	cup sunflower seeds, pumpkin seeds, or nuts
2	Tablespoons vinaigrette dressing

DIRECTIONS:

1. Combine salad ingredients in a big bowl. Toss well.
2. Add dressing.

2211 MEAL PLAN SERVINGS

Add ½ cup (about 1 ounce) whole-grain crackers to make the meal

2	1 cup greens + 1 cup chopped veggies
2	½ cup edamame + ¼ cup seeds or nuts
1	½ cup whole-grain crackers
1	salad dressing/seeds or nuts

Brown Rice, Chickpea, and Veggie Bowl

Makes 2 servings

Ever wonder what to do with leftover rice or pasta? Try this fast meal that's got everything you need in one bowl. I chop the broccoli first and steam it for 1 to 2 minutes in a microwavable bowl, covered with a little water. During that time, I chop the other veggies. This tasty meal is ready to go in less than 5 minutes. Try adding one of the homemade vinaigrettes or the peanut sauce (recipe later in this section) to add a burst of flavor.

INGREDIENTS:

1	cup cooked brown rice, pasta, or other grain
2	cups canned chickpeas, drained and rinsed
2	cups chopped cooked broccoli
1	cup chopped red (or any color) peppers
1	cup chopped tomatoes
4	Tablespoons crumbled feta cheese
2	Tablespoons vinaigrette dressing

DIRECTIONS:

1. For each serving, place half the brown rice, chickpeas, broccoli, and peppers in a large individual bowl, each in their own spot.
2. Top each bowl with tomatoes, feta, and dressing.

2211 MEAL PLAN SERVINGS

2	2 cups broccoli, peppers, and tomatoes
2	1 cup chickpeas + 2 Tablespoons feta cheese
1	½ cup cooked brown rice
1	1 Tablespoon dressing

Super Salad in a Jar

Makes 2 servings

Mason jar salads are so easy to make, plus they last up to three days in the fridge. Layer this way: salad dressing, chopped veggies or fruits, cooked grains, proteins, greens, and nuts and seeds last. This recipe is just a guideline. Be creative, adding any ingredients you have on hand in the order listed. If you've got a few minutes to wait for your dinner to cook, that's the perfect time to make tomorrow's mason jar salad!

INGREDIENTS:

4	Tablespoons of your favorite salad dressing
2	cups finely chopped carrots
1	cup cooked barley, brown rice, or quinoa (or any grain)
1	cup chopped grilled chicken breast or other protein of your choice
2	cups mixed greens
4	Tablespoons slivered almonds

DIRECTIONS:

1. Divide the ingredients in the order listed between 2 24-ounce Mason jars.
2. When ready to eat, turn the jar upside down to mix the salad ingredients with the dressing.

2211 MEAL PLAN SERVINGS

2	carrots and greens
2	chicken and almonds
1	½ cup cooked grain
1	salad dressing and almonds

Turkey, Cheese, and Pesto Roll

Makes 2 servings

You can personalize this quick and easy recipe any way you like, adding or substituting your favorite proteins, such as hummus, veggie "meat" slices, chicken, roast beef, or ham. The pesto gives the roll a zing of flavor. I like to prepare these ahead of time and take them with me when traveling as a fast lunch option.

INGREDIENTS:

4	ounces sliced turkey breast
2	mozzarella cheese sticks
2	teaspoons prepared pesto
2	small whole-grain wraps or tortillas

DIRECTIONS:

1. Spread the pesto on the wraps or tortillas.
2. Roll 2 ounces of turkey slices around one cheese stick and place at the edge of the wrap or tortilla.
3. Roll up the wrap or tortilla tightly.

2211 MEAL PLAN SERVINGS

Add 1 cup pepper slices and 1 apple to make a meal

2	1 cup pepper slices + 1 apple
2	2 ounces turkey + 1 ounce cheese (3 ounces)
1	1 tortilla or small wrap
1	1 teaspoon pesto

Hummus Pocket

Makes 2 servings

INGREDIENTS:

1½	cups prepared hummus
2	cups shredded dark lettuce, cabbage, or other greens
8	grape tomatoes, sliced
4	Tablespoons diced olives
1	whole wheat pita

DIRECTIONS:

1. Cut the pita in half.
2. Spread half the hummus in each pita pocket.
3. Top each half with greens, tomatoes, and olives.

2211 MEAL PLAN SERVINGS

Add 1 cup canned peaches to make a meal

2	greens and tomatoes + 1 cup canned peaches
2	¾ cup hummus
1	half of a whole grain pita bread
1	hummus/olives

Slow Cooker Lentil and Veggie Soup

Makes 12 1-cup servings

This recipe is a go-to when it's time to stock the freezer with a hearty soup. I like to divide the soup into three containers: one to eat right away and two to freeze for another time. Each serving provides a perfect mix of produce and protein and is loaded with fiber. Choose red, yellow, brown, green, or black lentils—your choice. You can use frozen chopped onions and prechopped carrots and celery for a time-saver.

INGREDIENTS:

1	medium onion, chopped
3	cloves garlic, finely chopped (or 3 teaspoons minced garlic or ½ teaspoon garlic powder)
2	cups chopped celery
2	cups chopped carrots
½	teaspoon salt
½	teaspoon pepper
1	Tablespoon Italian seasoning
1½	cups dry lentils (red, brown, yellow, or green), rinsed
1	15-ounce can diced tomatoes
8	cups vegetable stock
2	bay leaves
6	cups chopped fresh spinach (or 1 cup frozen chopped spinach or greens)
1	teaspoon red wine vinegar

DIRECTIONS:

1. Place all ingredients except the spinach and red wine vinegar in a 6-quart slow cooker. Stir well.
2. Cook on high for 5 hours, or until lentils and veggies are soft.
3. Remove bay leaves.
4. Add the spinach and red wine vinegar.
5. Stir well before serving.

2211 MEAL PLAN SERVINGS

Add 1 side salad with 1 Tablespoon Italian dressing and 1/2 whole-wheat pita to make a meal

2	veggies in the soup + side salad
2	lentils in the soup
1	1/2 pita
1	dressing on the salad

Tofu, Broccoli, and Sweet Potato Bowl

Makes 4 servings

What kind of spice are you in the mood for? Is it African, Indian, Italian, or Greek? This recipe is simple, easy to make, and can be tweaked to meet your taste. Add extra veggies if you have them around to boost this bowl of flavor even more!

INGREDIENTS:

1	package extra-firm tofu (14 to 16 ounces)
4	cups fresh chopped broccoli
2	medium sweet potatoes
2	Tablespoons olive oil or avocado oil
1	Tablespoon spice mix of your choice (African, Indian, Italian, Greek)
½	teaspoon garlic salt
½	cup chopped peanuts (or any nuts)

DIRECTIONS:

1. Preheat the oven to 425 degrees.
2. Wrap the tofu in a clean kitchen towel or paper towels and set on a plate. Cover with a heavy pan. Drain off water in the sink.
3. Wash and peel the sweet potatoes. Cut into small chunks.
4. Toss the sweet potatoes with ½ Tablespoon of olive oil.
5. Cut tofu into bite-size pieces and place in a medium bowl.
6. Add seasoning mix and 1 Tablespoon of oil. Mix well to coat the tofu.
7. In another medium bowl, mix the broccoli, ½ Tablespoon of oil, and garlic salt.
8. Line two baking sheet pans with foil and spray with cooking spray or use nonstick pans.

9. Spread the tofu on one pan and the sweet potato chunks and broccoli on the second pan.
10. Bake for 15 minutes. Turn the tofu, broccoli, and sweet potatoes and bake for 15 more minutes, or until they begin to brown.
11. Divide the sweet potatoes, tofu, and broccoli evenly into four bowls.
12. Sprinkle with chopped peanuts.

2211 MEAL PLAN SERVINGS

Add 1 cup melon slices to make a meal

2	1 cup broccoli + 1 cup sliced melon
2	¼ block of tofu + 2 Tablespoons peanuts
1	½ of a medium sweet potato (about ½ cup)
1	oil and peanuts

Dinners

Citrus Salmon

Makes 4 servings

This salmon recipe goes well with simple steamed broccoli and brown rice. The combination of orange and lemon and added spice complements the salmon. This recipe works well with any fish you enjoy. If you don't have a zester, use a grater. If there is no grater, chop the orange rind into very small pieces. This is a go-to recipe in our home.

INGREDIENTS:

1	pound salmon filets (fresh or frozen)
1	orange
1	lemon
½	teaspoon salt
½	teaspoon pepper
2	teaspoons avocado or olive oil
2	Tablespoons brown sugar
1	Tablespoon chili powder
1	garlic clove, chopped, or ¼ teaspoon garlic powder

DIRECTIONS:

1. Zest the orange.
2. Juice the orange and the lemon. Combine juices with salt and pepper in a shallow baking dish.
3. Add salmon filets. Marinate for 20 minutes or longer in the refrigerator, turning several times.
4. Preheat the oven to 425 degrees.
5. Coat a sheet pan with foil and 1 teaspoon of oil.

6. In a small dish, combine the orange zest, brown sugar, chili powder, and garlic.
7. Place the salmon on the baking sheet skin-side down and rub the orange zest mixture over the top of the salmon.
8. Drizzle 1 teaspoon of oil over the salmon.
9. Bake for 15-18 minutes or until salmon is flaky.

2211 MEAL PLAN SERVINGS

Add 1 sliced orange and ½ cup cooked brown rice to make a meal

2	1 cup steamed broccoli and 1 sliced orange
2	1 serving salmon
1	½ cup cooked brown rice
1	oil and salmon

Lisa's Slow Cooker Chicken Chili

Makes 8 servings

This simple chili with a kick of flavor has been in my friend Lisa's family for as long as she can remember. It works great when you're in need of a hearty meal, or if you have friends or family coming over for dinner. If you're in a hurry, place ingredients in a large pot on the stove, heat to medium, and cook for 20 minutes, stirring frequently. You can use rotisserie chicken or canned chicken if you prefer. Topping ideas: diced tomatoes, chopped avocados, salsa, sour cream, or plain Greek yogurt

INGREDIENTS:

3	cups cooked chicken, cut into bite-size pieces (about 2 breasts) or 4 5-ounce cans of cooked chicken
2	16-ounce cans great northern beans (with liquid)
1	16-ounce jar picante sauce or salsa
1	8-ounce block of pepper jack cheese, cut into chunks
1	Tablespoon ground cumin

DIRECTIONS:

1. Place all ingredients in a slow cooker.
2. Cook on low for 3 hours.
3. Add toppings and enjoy!

2211 MEAL PLAN SERVINGS

Add 1 cup corn tortilla chips, 1 cup pineapple, 1 cup carrot sticks, and avocado slices to make a meal

2	1 cup pineapple + 1 cup carrot sticks
2	1 cup chili
1	1 cup corn tortilla chips
1	avocado slices

Fast Fried Rice

Makes 4 servings

This is an easy "What do I make for dinner?" solution everyone always enjoys. It works well with any leftover veggies you have, or if your greens are on their last few days in the fridge. I keep bags of frozen mixed veggies on hand just for this dish. It's also a real cost-saver—and eggs provide ample high-quality protein.

INGREDIENTS:

8	eggs
3	green onions, chopped
1	12-ounce bag (about 3 cups) frozen mixed vegetables (peas, carrots, green beans)
4	cups fresh chopped greens (kale, spinach, bok choy) or 1 cup frozen chopped greens
1	Tablespoon (3 teaspoons) canola oil
¼	cup light soy sauce
1	teaspoon chopped fresh or dried ginger
2	cups cooked brown or white rice

DIRECTIONS:

1. In a medium bowl, scramble eggs.
2. In a large skillet, heat 1 teaspoon of oil on medium heat for 1 minute.
3. Add the eggs and scramble for 2 to 3 minutes, or until cooked. Set the eggs aside on a plate.
4. Heat the remaining 2 teaspoons of oil on medium heat for 30 seconds.
5. Add the chopped onions and greens, and sauté for 1 to 2 minutes.

6. Meanwhile, microwave the mixed vegetables for 3 minutes.
7. Add veggies to the pan and cook for 2 to 3 minutes.
8. Stir in the cooked eggs and rice.
9. Mix in the soy sauce and ginger and cook on low for 2 minutes, stirring frequently.

2211 MEAL PLAN SERVINGS

2	2 cups veggies
2	2 eggs
1	½ cup rice
1	oil and eggs

Veg Out Pizza

Makes 4 servings

Whether you use an inexpensive frozen thin-crust pizza or you make your own crust or purchase premade pizza dough, this pizza with a boost of veggies will be a hit. Load it up with any veggies you have on hand. You can add extra protein (chopped chicken, ham, bacon, sausage, or veggie sausage) if you like.

INGREDIENTS:

1	small frozen thin crust pizza of your choice
2	cups chopped onions, peppers, broccoli, mushrooms (or any veggies you have in the refrigerator)
4	cups fresh kale or spinach (or other greens) or 1 cup frozen greens
2	teaspoons avocado, olive, or canola oil
1	cup shredded low-fat mozzarella cheese
1	teaspoon pizza seasoning

DIRECTIONS:

1. Wash and chop veggies.
2. Preheat the oven to 425 degrees.
3. Add the oil to a large skillet and heat on medium for 1 minute.
4. Add veggies and sauté for 2 to 3 minutes or until soft.
5. Add greens and sauté for 1 to 2 minutes or until cooked down.
6. Spread the veggies on the pizza.
7. Sprinkle pizza seasoning and shredded cheese over the pizza.
8. Bake according to directions or until the cheese is lightly browned, about 12 to 15 minutes.

2211 MEAL PLAN SERVINGS

Add 1 cup mixed berries to make a meal

2	veggies and spinach + mixed berries
2	shredded cheese and cheese/meat pizza
1	pizza crust
1	oil

Tilapia with Tomato-Basil Salsa and Roasted Potatoes

Makes 4 servings

I'm always looking for fast, tasty fish recipes that are easy to make and low cost. This recipe uses tilapia because it's widely available in most supermarkets, but choose any whitefish you enjoy. Roasted potatoes are one of my favorite sides, as they're loaded with nutrients, cost-effective, and so tasty. The lemony tomato-basil salsa tops off this meal perfectly.

INGREDIENTS:

2	cups diced fresh potatoes (about 2 large)
½	teaspoon salt
1	pound frozen tilapia (or other whitefish) filets, fresh or frozen
1	lemon, zested
⅛	teaspoon pepper
1	pint (2 cups) grape or cherry tomatoes
¼	cup fresh chopped basil (or 1 teaspoon dried basil)
2	teaspoons avocado, olive, or canola oil
1	medium garlic clove, minced (or 1 teaspoon minced garlic in a jar or ¼ teaspoon garlic powder)

DIRECTIONS:

1. Preheat the oven to 375 degrees.
2. Line a sheet pan with foil and spray with cooking spray or use a nonstick pan.
3. In a medium bowl, mix diced potatoes with 1 teaspoon oil. Place on the baking sheet. Sprinkle with ¼ teaspoon salt.

4. Bake diced potatoes for 15 minutes.
5. Line a second baking sheet with foil or a baking mat. Spray with cooking spray.
6. Place the fish on the baking sheet. Squeeze the juice from half of the lemon on the fish. Top with ¼ teaspoon salt and ¼ teaspoon pepper.
7. Bake the fish and potatoes for 15 additional minutes.
8. Meanwhile, prepare the salsa. Slice the tomatoes in half. In a medium bowl, mix tomatoes, basil, 1 teaspoon olive oil, garlic, the juice from the other half of the lemon, and ½ teaspoon of grated lemon zest.
9. Remove the tilapia and potatoes from the oven. Potatoes should be tender, and fish should be flaky.
10. Divide tilapia and potatoes evenly onto four plates. Top the tilapia with homemade salsa.

2211 MEAL PLAN SERVINGS

Add a side salad with homemade vinaigrette

2	salsa and a side salad
2	tilapia
1	½ cup potatoes
1	oil; vinaigrette dressing

Cinnamon Fruit Salad

Makes 4 servings

I've been making this cinnamon fruit salad ever since I became a Registered Dietitian and learned about the magic of adding a little orange juice (high in vitamin C) to cut fruit to keep it from browning. I love the burst of extra spice from the cinnamon. You can use any combination of fruit you have on hand, but I love this mix because of the bright colors and fresh flavor.

INGREDIENTS:

1	cup grapes
1	cup blueberries
1	cup pineapple, cut into bite-size pieces
1	medium orange, cut into bite-size pieces
1	apple, cut into bite-size pieces
½	cup orange juice
1	teaspoon cinnamon

DIRECTIONS:

1. Wash fruit.
2. Add fruit to a medium bowl and toss with orange juice.
3. Sprinkle with cinnamon and mix well.

2211 MEAL PLAN SERVINGS

Add burgers/buns, carrot sticks, and grilled asparagus basted with olive oil to make a meal

2	1 cup fruit salad and 1 cup carrot sticks
2	burger/veggie burger
1	whole grain bun
1	olive oil

Slow Cooker Sausage and Veggie Pasta

Makes 12 1-cup servings

Having guests for dinner or feeding a large family? This is a "make it and forget it" recipe that's ready in three hours. I like using turkey sausage but choose any sausage you like best in this recipe. Whole-grain spaghetti or pasta works well. It provides extra fiber while coming out soft and chewy, simply perfect for a slow cooker dish. The extra veggies add a burst of flavor and bolster the nutritional value of this tasty dish. One serving provides a complete 2211 meal. If you're in a hurry, bake this recipe on 350 degrees in a 9 X 13-inch pan covered for 1 hour.

INGREDIENTS:

2	teaspoons avocado, olive, or canola oil
1	pound low-fat Italian sausage, crumbled or sliced
1	medium onion, chopped
2	red (or any color) peppers, coarsely chopped (about 2 cups)
1	Tablespoon Italian seasoning
1	15-ounce can petite diced tomatoes (regular or fire-roasted)
1	28-ounce jar red pasta sauce
3	cups low-fat cottage cheese
1	cup shredded low-fat mozzarella cheese
½	pound (½ box) whole-grain spaghetti or pasta
1	10-ounce package frozen spinach

DIRECTIONS:

1. In a large skillet, heat oil on medium for 30 seconds. Add sausage. Brown for 3 to 4 minutes. Drain if needed.
2. Add onions and peppers to the skillet. Cook for 3 additional minutes.
3. Take the skillet off heat and add Italian seasoning, diced tomatoes, and pasta sauce and combine well.
4. In a medium bowl, stir together cottage cheese and ½ cup of the shredded mozzarella cheese. Reserve the remaining mozzarella to top the dish.
5. Spray the interior of the slow cooker with cooking spray.
6. Pour ⅓ of the turkey/veggie/sauce mix into the slow cooker and spread evenly.
7. Top with ⅓ of the uncooked spaghetti or pasta, breaking to fit.
8. Spread ⅓ of the cheese mixture over the pasta.
9. Spread ⅓ of the spinach over the cheese.
10. Repeat the layers two more times.
11. Cook on high for 3 hours.
12. Sprinkle the remaining ½ cup of shredded mozzarella on top.

2211 MEAL PLAN SERVINGS

2	2 cups veggies/sauce
2	sausage, cottage cheese, and cheese (2 ounces)
1	½ cup cooked pasta
1	oil

Sauces and
Dressings

Peanut Sauce

Makes 8 2-Tablespoon servings

This peanut sauce adds just the right flavor to steamed veggies, meal bowls, noodle dishes, and grilled tofu or chicken. It also works great as a dipping sauce for veggies or steamed dumplings. Make this ahead and keep it in the refrigerator for up to two weeks. Add warm water to thin, if needed.

INGREDIENTS:

½	cup creamy peanut butter
2	Tablespoons light soy sauce
2	Tablespoons honey
1	Tablespoon rice vinegar or lime juice
½	teaspoon garlic powder
1	teaspoon spicy sweet red chili sauce (more if you like it extra spicy!)
4	Tablespoons warm water

DIRECTIONS:

1. Whisk all ingredients (except for water) together in a small bowl.
2. When well blended, add the warm water, 1 Tablespoon at a time, to desired thickness.
3. Store in a sealed container in the refrigerator for up to 2 weeks.

Basic Balsamic Vinaigrette

Makes 10 1-Tablespoon servings

Freshly made salad dressing is easy to prepare and adds so much flavor to fresh greens. This dressing is a family favorite and tastes great.

INGREDIENTS:

¼	cup balsamic vinegar
⅓	cup olive oil or avocado oil (or your favorite oil)
1	teaspoon maple syrup or honey
2	teaspoons Dijon mustard
1	teaspoon chopped garlic (or 1 teaspoon minced garlic in a jar or ½ teaspoon garlic powder)
½	teaspoon salt
¼	teaspoon black pepper

In a jar with a tight lid, combine all ingredients. Shake to combine. Refrigerate and use within two weeks.

Lemony Herb Vinaigrette

Makes 12 1-Tablespoon servings

This refreshing salad dressing is so versatile. Choose your favorite fresh or dried herbs to add new flavors.

INGREDIENTS:

½	cup olive oil or avocado oil (or your favorite oil)
¼	cup lemon juice (juice of 1 lemon)
1	Tablespoon fresh or dried herbs (try dried Italian herb mix or a mix of basil, tarragon, parsley, and dill)
1	garlic clove, minced (or 1 teaspoon minced garlic in a jar or ½ teaspoon garlic powder)
1	teaspoon Dijon mustard
½	teaspoon salt
¼	teaspoon black pepper

In a jar with a tight lid, combine all ingredients. Shake to combine. Store in the refrigerator and use within two weeks.

PART II

How to MOVE

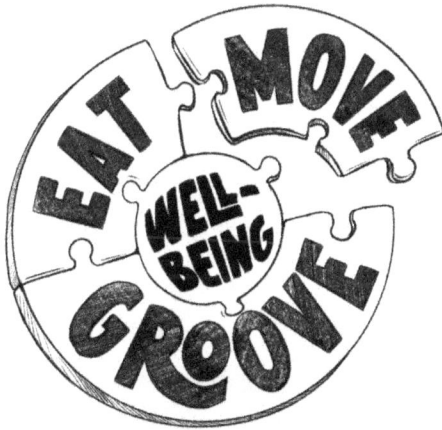

8

How to MOVE:
The 2211 MOVE Framework

To maintain health, enhance well-being, and get the most out of life, we need to move our bodies. The simple, sensible 2211 framework helps you learn to move in ways that feel good to you, energize you, and keep you strong and able to do the things you want to do every day.

Use the three pillars of the 2211 MOVE foundation to get yourself moving at least 33 minutes a day on most days:

- Purposefully move your body in ways you enjoy that get your heart beating deeper and faster than usual (aerobic exercise) for at least 22 minutes a day.

- Do strength, stability, and stretching activities for at least 11 minutes a day.

- Get up and move often during the day.

22 ‖ 11

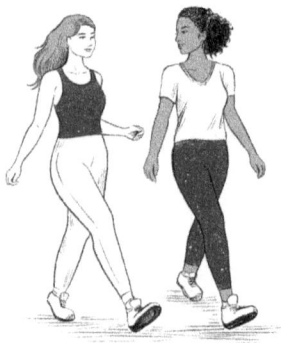

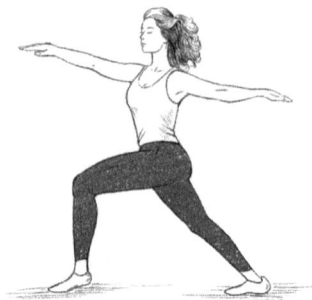

With the **22**11 MOVE plan, you decide how you want to move your body, what feels good to you, and what you enjoy doing. Your activities might include walking, biking, swimming, golf, basketball, or pickleball. You can also build movement into your day while you get things done.

"I walk to get something done. I live my life by walking to get groceries, fill my backpack with ten pounds of food, and walk home," says Carol Kennedy-Armbruster, PhD, teaching professor emeritus with Indiana University, Bloomington, and the co-author of *Fitness and Well-Being for Life*. You might carry laundry up and down stairs, wash windows, or clean the house to be active.

Kennedy-Armbruster notes that everyday activities based around your family can also fit into the **22**11 MOVE plan and keep us strong. "Lifting my grandchild helps me improve what I need to do. As my grandchild grows, I lift more weight." That's a natural progression of training our bodies to lift more weight.

The key is to investigate what works for you and remember to be flexible. Perhaps you lift hand weights, or jugs of water.

The key is to give your body something (or someone) to lift to help strengthen you.

Just as we have love foods in the EAT plan, it's important to move your body in ways you love to move—in ways that bring you joy. That will be different for each of us.

First, find activities you enjoy doing. That may sound too simple, but we'll continue moving our bodies day after day if we enjoy the movement and feel good doing it.

Take it from exercise physiologist Ann Swartz, PhD, co-director of the Physical Activity and Health Research Lab at the University of Wisconsin–Milwaukee. Her best advice: "If we enjoy what we're doing, we're going to stick with it." Swartz encourages people to "figure out where you find joy in your movement." This is the key to maintaining an active lifestyle over a lifetime.

What do you like to do?

Do you enjoy dancing? It's a wonderful way to move to music. How about joining a Zumba class or taking adult tap lessons? Maybe you'd enjoy dancing at home to your favorite music—by yourself or with a friend or partner.

What did you enjoy doing as a kid? Maybe it's time to get back to playing like we did as children. Engaging in play is also a key component of finding our groove. Running around and playing (and laughing) provides you with a whole host of benefits.

How do you like to do these activities? Do you enjoy moving by yourself, with a friend or loved one, with your pets, or in a group?

What time of day do you enjoy moving your body? Do you enjoy moving in the morning, during the middle of the day, or in the evening? Are you a morning person or a night owl?

Where do you like to move? Outside? Inside? In nature? On city sidewalks? Walking on the soft grass or a hiking trail? While talking with friends?

If you have a favorite activity you enjoy doing most days, what are one or two other activities you also enjoy? If you enjoy walking outdoors but the weather is really bad, or if you just want a change, what's your fallback activity? Can you walk in the local mall instead? Or go to an exercise class at your local Y?

What do you like to eat and drink before, during, or after you move your body? Having these foods and drinks ready and accessible can help you move more and feel better during and after your exercise.

Make sure to consider any aches and pains you have and your current health conditions. Do you have physical limitations, such as an arthritic knee, that impact how you can move your body? If so, how can you still move within these limitations? What assistance can support your movement? Water aerobics, warm water exercise classes, or chair yoga may be great options.

22 Minutes of Heart-Pumping Movement

Aerobic activities get your heart beating and make you breathe more deeply—bike riding, brisk walking, or exercising to a video, for example. You might prefer 22 minutes or more of activity at one time or you might find it more convenient to get your movement in short bursts—by going up and down stairs a few times, or vacuuming at a steady pace, for example. Or you might prefer a brisk walk with a family member, friend, or dog—or all three.

Other aerobic activity examples include these:

- Dancing
- Zumba or other exercise class
- Jogging
- Rowing

- Kayaking
- Hiking up and down hills or walking in the water
- Swimming
- Bicycling
- Mowing the lawn with a mower you push
- Mopping the floor
- Playing table tennis
- Walking briskly to the store or bus stop
- Playing pickleball or tennis

11 Minutes of Strengthening, Stability, and Stretching

Strength, stability, and stretching activities are exercises or movements that strengthen your muscles and bones and keep you flexible. They help you move easily, function well, and avoid falls and injury. Adding exercises that help you maintain balance can help prevent falls and injuries.

You can aim for 11 minutes or more of these activities all at once (such as taking a strength class at your local wellness center) or by adding in short strength and flexibility breaks during the day. Some of these activities include the following:

- Standing up and sitting down 10 times in a row
- Lifting boxes or groceries
- Gardening, especially digging in the dirt
- Raking leaves
- Using resistance bands for strength exercises
- Using hand weights for strength exercises
- Doing lunges while walking
- Doing toe stands
- Balancing on one leg at a time
- Doing sit-ups or push-ups
- Yoga

- Tai chi
- Qigong
- Pilates
- Paddle boarding
- Water exercise classes
- Household chores such as doing laundry, doing dishes, cleaning, washing windows, vacuuming

Some activities you enjoy provide benefits for your cardiovascular health and strength at the same time. For example, when you swim, pushing against the water with your arms and kicking help build strength, while the activity makes your heart beat faster and makes you breathe more heavily. When you bicycle or walk briskly up and down stairs or up hills, you're strengthening your leg muscles while also gaining cardiovascular benefits.

Move Throughout the Day

Move often throughout the day, getting up at least once an hour to walk, stretch, or take movement breaks from sedentary work at a computer or TV watching. That may be as simple as making phone calls while walking, getting the mail, or playing with your dog for a five-minute break. There are many ways you can move throughout the day:

- Prepare a meal or snack
- Walk through the office to meet with a colleague instead of emailing or texting
- Take lunch outside
- Walk up and down a few flights of stairs
- Listen to a short podcast while walking
- Walk to get a cup of tea
- Power clean a bathroom

- Vacuum, sweep, or mop the floor
- Start a load of laundry or hang clothes out to dry
- Choose a job where you move a lot during the day

Exercise with Others

You may enjoy exercising more when you exercise with others. You can catch up, share experiences, and laugh. Plus, you may be more consistent when you're relying on a friend, family member, or exercise group (and they're relying on you) to stay active. It keeps you accountable to yourself and others, which can be very motivating.

Exercising in community with friends, family members, or even strangers is one important way to be social and enjoy the company of others. This is helpful for decreasing loneliness and depression. We take care of others when we move with them, including our pets. Everyone benefits.

Exercising with others in a group setting offers other benefits too. Planning ahead to attend group exercise classes, scheduled pickleball matches, yoga classes, or walking groups helps you prioritize moving your body in ways you enjoy with others. When you block out time in your day to stay active, you're much more apt to be consistent with exercising.

2211 MOVE Sample Days

Check out these examples of options for implementing the 2211 MOVE plan in two sample days. You can enjoy movement with friends, accomplishing household tasks, or enjoying the outdoors. You may prefer to move your body for exercise early in the day, in the middle of the day, or later in the day. It's up to you. Be creative and build in activities you enjoy each day.

Sample Day 1

- **Morning:** Brisk walk for 22 minutes (22 minutes of heart-pumping movement)
- **Afternoon:** 6 minutes of strength exercises using resistance bands while listening to your favorite music (6 of 11 minutes of strength, stretching, and stability)
- **Evening:** 5 minutes of stretching, one-leg stands, and balance exercises (5 of 11 minutes of strength, stretching, and stability)
- **During the day:** Walk or move around for 5 minutes once every hour during the day for a break. Accomplish a task; take your dog or children for a walk.

Sample Day 2

- **Morning:** 11 minutes of online yoga (11 minutes of strength, stretching, and stability)
- **Afternoon:** 11 minutes of a walk break while listening to a book or podcast (11 of 22 minutes of heart-pumping exercise)
- **After dinner:** 11 minutes of a brisk walk around the block with your family or friends (11 minutes of heart-pumping exercise)
- **During the day:** Walk or move around for 5 minutes once every hour during the day for a break. Have a walking meeting with a friend or colleague if you're at work.

MOVEMENT TERMS EXPLAINED

Physical activity: Any movement that involves your muscles and expends energy. Physical activity can be any type of movement: moving around your home doing chores, walking, playing sports or exercising.

Exercise: Physical activity that is planned, structured, and repetitive, designed to maintain or boost your fitness and health.

Cardiovascular exercise: Exercise that raises your heart rate and makes you breathe harder—you can talk while doing it, but you can't sing. Brisk walking, jogging, going up and down stairs, and similar activities are all ways to get cardiovascular exercise. Also known as aerobic exercise.

Strength exercise: Exercise that requires your muscles to work harder than usual. Strength work usually includes external resistance, such as weights, exercise bands, or even your own body weight. Also called resistance training.

Stability exercise: Exercise that helps to maintain or strengthen joint stability or improve balance.

Stretching exercise: Exercise that moves joints and groups of joints through their full range of motion.

Getting Started

If you're not used to moving much, build up to 33 minutes a day gradually. Your goal is 22 or more minutes a day of purposeful movement where your heart is pumping and you are breathing deeper and more often than normal (cardiovascular exercise) and 11 minutes a day or more of movement that strengthens, stretches, and stabilizes your body.

You might not be able to move at this level when you first start. Stick with it. Start with easier movement for a shorter time, then add a bit more every few days until you're up to 33 minutes in total. Don't overdo it and give yourself a day off now and then. You may get up to 33 minutes a day within a few weeks. When you feel ready, you might add more time or change up your activities to keep things interesting. It's totally up to you.

Akin to how we eat, how we move makes an impact on our health and well-being by what we do over weeks, months, and years. Our bodies respond to how we move over time. You may not move as much as you'd like every day, but some movement is better than none. When life gets in the way and you have other concerns to attend to, your exercise time may be limited. If you can move your body most days utilizing the 2211 framework, you'll be caring for your health and well-being and you'll feel good too.

Benefits of Being Physically Active

In addition to boosting our physical health and fitness, moving our bodies does amazing things for us:

- We feel better when we're active.
- We're more energized when we move our bodies. That feeling stays with us all day, not just when we're active.
- We get a boost in our mood and feel less stressed when we're active.
- We can handle the activities of daily living more easily, such as picking up a toddler or carrying groceries.
- Better strength and balance help prevent falls and injuries.

It's Your Choice

How you move your body is up to you. The key is to find movements and activities you enjoy and that you can easily build into your day. When you're consistent with moving your body, you'll feel good, enjoy what you do, and reap the benefits for your health and well-being.

Your MOVE plan won't be the same as anyone else's. Your plan is built around your day, the activities you like to do, your commitments and obligations, where you live, what's accessible to you each day, and many other factors. Be flexible and creative to make your MOVE plan work for you so that you're empowered to move every day. And remember, focus on movements you enjoy so you will move simply as a part of your day.

9

The 2211 MOVE Plan

Now that you understand the framework of the MOVE plan, let's explore how the recommendation for the daily 22 or more minutes of heart-pumping movement and the 11 minutes or more of strength, stability, and stretching movement came about. Then let's find simple ways to build movement into your day.

In the same way we make it easy to nourish our bodies with highly nutritious foods by planning, grocery shopping, and keeping optimal choices available to us, we can set up and reinforce movement opportunities throughout the day and make exercise easy. We may *know* how to eat well and move our bodies for optimal health and well-being, but *doing* it is the key.

First, let's get a bit more background on the science behind MOVE.

Movement Research and Guidelines

The MOVE recommendations for the 2211 simple lifestyle plan originated from the *Physical Activity Guidelines for Americans*, released in 2018. These national goals for activity provide guidance to help maintain or improve health through physical activity.

The guidelines are a joint effort of the Centers for Disease Control and Prevention (CDC), the National Institutes of Health, and the President's Council on Sports, Fitness, & Nutrition.

The guidelines for adults include these key points:

- Move more and sit less throughout the day. Some physical activity is better than none. Adults who sit less and do any amount of moderate to vigorous physical activity gain some health benefits.

- For substantial health benefits, do at least 150 minutes to 300 minutes a week of moderate aerobic physical activity, or 75 minutes to 150 minutes a week of vigorous aerobic activity—or a mix of both (that's 22 minutes a day or more of moderate aerobic activity).

- Aerobic activity should be spread throughout the week whenever possible.

- Additional health benefits are gained by going beyond 300 minutes of moderate intensity physical activity a week.

- Moderate to vigorous muscle-strengthening activities that involve all major muscle groups two or more days a week give you additional health benefits (that equates to 11 minutes a day of strength activities).

The American College of Sports Medicine, a worldwide leader in exercise and sports medicine, also provides helpful guidelines for staying active:

- All healthy adults aged 18 to 65 years should participate in moderate intensity aerobic physical activity for a minimum of 30 minutes on five days per week, or vigorous intensity aerobic activity for a minimum of 20 minutes on three days per week.
- Every adult should perform activities that maintain or increase muscular strength and endurance for a minimum of two days per week.

Additional recommendations for MOVE that reinforce these guidelines come from the American Heart Association, the American Cancer Society, and the American College of Lifestyle Medicine. Recommendations from the American Diabetes Association include regular movement breaks to help with blood glucose control. Even 10 (or 11) minutes of activity at one time is beneficial for overall health.

MOVE with the 2211 Plan

We know that moving on a consistent basis makes us feel better, boosts our mood, offers opportunities to be social, lowers the risk for disease, keeps us fit and strong, and helps us in countless other ways. Let's make it simple. That's where the 2211 plan really helps. Each day is based on 22 minutes of purposeful movement that boosts your heart rate and gets you breathing heavier than normal, and 11 minutes of strength, stretching, or stability movement.

The **22**11 MOVE lifestyle plan combines the latest research and recommendations into a simple, doable, daily plan. You can easily bring the MOVE plan into your life:

- MOVE at least **22** minutes a day in a way that boosts your heart rate and gets you breathing more heavily (aerobic activity) per day. That's equal to at least 154 minutes per week.

- MOVE at least **11** minutes a day doing strength/stretching/stability activities. That's equal to at least 77 minutes per week.

- MOVE often during the day, getting up at least once an hour to walk, stretch, or take a movement break.

According to the CDC, only about one-quarter of adults ages 18 and over met the exercise recommendations for both aerobic and strengthening in 2020. As we get older, Americans become increasingly sedentary. For men, 41 percent met the guidelines in the 18 to 34 age group, with decreases to 29 percent (for ages 35 to 49), and 21 percent (for those who are 50 to 64). By age 65 and older, only 15 percent of Americans meet the recommendations. While 28 percent of women met the guidelines in the 18 to 34 age group, that dropped to 22 percent (in the 35 to 49 age group), and 17 percent (among people who are 50 to 64). Only 10 percent of women meet the recommendations at age 65 and older.

Increased Lifespan and Health Span

Staying active is associated with a longer health span, or the number of years we live in good health to optimize the quality of life. It's not just about living longer; it's about living longer and being healthy during those additional years. That means maximizing our years by maintaining optimal physical, mental, and emotional health so we can enjoy life to the fullest.

A recent study that followed over 116,000 people for more than thirty years found that compared to those who did little or no physical activity, those who were moderately active (from 150 to 300 minutes a week) enhanced their longevity by 20 percent. That's the difference between living to age 70 or living to age 84. That's the real power of moving your body.

As we go through life, staying active, strong, flexible, and social becomes even more important. We want to be moving more, not less, as we age—and we want to interact with others who move more too. Moving is the foundation that helps maintain independence and the ability to enjoy life. We need simple, easy, low-stress ways to stay active as we age—and we need to enjoy doing them.

Small Increases = Big Results

In one recent study analyzing the activity of nearly 5,000 adults, small increases in physical activity were found to boost longevity. Adding only 10 minutes of moderate to vigorous physical activity a day made a significant difference in how long participants lived. The results were positive for everyone: women and men of all ethnic backgrounds. Increasing activity by 10 minutes per day boosted longevity by 7 percent. The benefit nearly doubled when activity was increased by 20 minutes a day.

Move Throughout the Day

Many studies have looked at the benefits of taking breaks from sitting. Less sitting and more movement during the day has been linked to a lower risk of many health problems, including anxiety, depression, Alzheimer's disease, cardiovascular disease, and type 2 diabetes. Plus, we just feel better when we move our bodies during the day.

In one study, sitting time and movement time were tracked for nearly 8,000 middle-aged and older adults. Over the course of four years, greater sitting time (being sedentary) and a longer duration of sedentary behavior (sitting for longer periods of time) were associated with decreases in longevity. Adults in the US are sedentary for an average of 9 to 10 hours per day, so there's plenty of opportunity to get up and move.

To make all this research practical, taking a five-minute movement break every hour over an eight-hour workday would meet the 33-minute goal for movement with the **2211 MOVE** plan. On busy days, plan five five-minute heart-pumping activity breaks and two five-minute strength breaks.

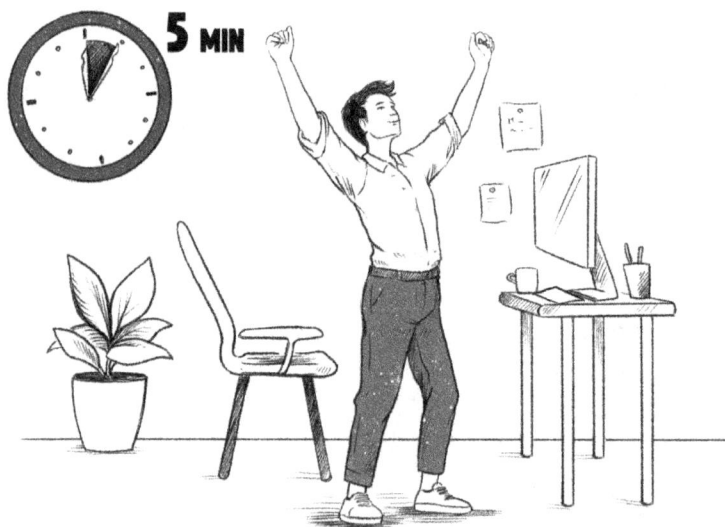

Move Five Minutes Each Hour

In 2023, researcher Keith Diaz, PhD, and his team at Columbia University reviewed self-reported movement data from over 13,000 listeners of National Public Radio's *The Body Electric* podcast. They found that the people who got up and moved for five minutes at least every hour during the day reported having more energy, better mood, and felt more engaged in their work, even with the movement interruptions.

The Bottom Line on Sitting Less and Moving More

The bottom line: Move frequently and more throughout the day. Break up sitting by moving for five or more minutes every hour during the day. You might set a timer as a reminder, plan tasks throughout the day to get up and move, schedule a walk with a friend or colleague, or make your dog incredibly happy by building in short walks throughout the day.

Benefits of Staying Strong

Maintaining strength, balance, and flexibility, especially as we get older, offers many amazing benefits. In a recent review of over 5,000 adults (nearly half women), Stuart Phillips, PhD, and his team of researchers from McMaster University in Canada reported that regularly participating in any resistance (strength) program will benefit adults and enhance health. Doing any strength exercise you can stay with consistently is beneficial and can help you stay stronger and increase mobility. Phillips notes that consistency is the key. Worry less about all the variables, such as whether machines or free weights are better. Simply find a place to get strong and do it consistently.

What if strength training is new to you? "Get some guidance on what exercises to do—and how to do them. Plan what you can commit to. If it's one day a week, that's better than zero days a week. If it's two days a week, that's better than one day a week. Find something you enjoy doing in an environment you enjoy doing it in, with people you enjoy being with," recommends Phillips.

Adding two 30-minute sessions of strength-based exercises each week can help you achieve this goal. Or, with the 2211 MOVE plan, the 11 means getting 11 minutes of strength or stability movement daily. Over a week, that's 77 minutes of strength-based activities, which meets and even exceeds the guidelines. You can find simple ways to build 11 minutes into your daily routine. You can even do just a minute or two at a time, or a couple of 5- to 6-minute strength breaks, or 11 minutes at once—whatever works for you that day.

The simplest strength and stability exercises use your own body weight to get stronger: Doing push-ups against a wall or getting up and down from a chair, for example. You might also use lightweight resistance bands.

If you prefer going to a gym, you can do strength training for 30 or more minutes twice a week with machines or free weights, or by attending a strength class. Going up and down stairs is a fantastic way to strengthen your legs while also getting cardiovascular benefits. No matter how you get your average of 11 minutes a day (or 60 to 77 minutes or more a week) in, activities that boost your strength and stability are core to the EAT MOVE GROOVE plan.

Just as we eat the rainbow by including a wide variety of fruits and vegetables, whole grains and starches, lean proteins, healthy fats, and love foods, we can apply the rainbow concept to MOVE. To do this, try new activities, change up your exercise routines, and include a wide variety of physical activities.

Good Things Happen When You MOVE

Loss of muscle mass and muscle function is one of the leading causes of falls, injuries, and, eventually, loss of independence. As we age, we lose muscle tissue and muscle function (sarcopenia). While to a degree this is a normal occurrence, we want to do everything possible to prevent or slow the decline. Implementing regular physical activity or movement into your day and consistently moving to strengthen your body is critical for decreasing the loss of muscle tissue and muscle function.

We also lose bone mass as a natural occurrence as we age (osteopenia and osteoporosis); thinner bones break easily. Here, too, we want to slow the loss. Optimal eating, balanced with physical activity, can decrease bone loss. When you have stronger bones, you have a lower risk of breaking them if you fall or are injured.

When you make the **2211 MOVE** program part of your well-being lifestyle, good things happen. According to Ann Swartz, PhD, from the University of Wisconsin–Milwaukee, "The list of all of the benefits of participating in exercise on a regular basis is endless."

- When we maintain an active lifestyle, we can simply do more. We can easily go about our daily life and physically do the things we want to do. That's a price-less gift.

- Staying active on a consistent basis plays an especially vital role in our emotional and mental health. When we feel better about ourselves by maintaining an active lifestyle, this can lower our risk of anxiety and depression.

- People who are physically active for approximately 150 minutes/week (at least 22 minutes a day) live longer and live with higher function than people who aren't physically active. That's what we want.

- Active people lower their risk of developing cardio-vascular disease, including heart attacks, strokes, and heart failure. Cardiovascular disease is the leading cause of death in the United States.

- Regular physical activity can lower blood pressure, blood cholesterol, and triglycerides.

- Regular physical activity lowers your risk of developing type 2 diabetes and helps control blood sugar levels if you're living with type 2 diabetes.

- Moving your body can decrease body fat and help you lose weight if that is one of your why goals. Staying active can also help you sustain weight loss.

- Regular physical activity can provide health benefits for people with osteoarthritis, osteoporosis, dementia, constipation, physical disabilities, and other conditions.

- Staying active with regular exercise may lower the risk of developing certain cancers, including bladder, breast, colon, endometrium, esophagus, kidney, lung, and stomach cancer. Cancer remains the second leading cause of death in the United States.

- Regular physical activity can enhance the quality of your sleep. Better sleep means better overall physical and mental well-being.

Take Inventory of Your MOVE Assets

To make moving more a part of your daily life, take inventory of your MOVE assets. You probably already have a lot of ways to make moving easier for you. For example, you may have comfortable clothing to exercise in, or running shoes or hiking boots in your closet. Access to the internet to find free exercise classes? How about friends or family members who would enjoy being active with you? Local parks or walking paths?

Stairs in your home? These are all MOVE assets that can help you stay active. Let's take a closer look at your MOVE inventory.

My MOVE Inventory

Personal Inventory

- ☐ Easy-to-move-in clothing
- ☐ Easy-to-move-in shoes
- ☐ My favorite music
- ☐ Pets to walk daily
- ☐ Friends and family to move with
- ☐ Friends and family to talk on the phone or videochat with while I move
- ☐ Colleagues to take walking breaks with at work

Equipment and Programs

- ☐ Hand weights
- ☐ Resistance bands
- ☐ Walking poles
- ☐ Fitness equipment such as a stationary bike or stepper
- ☐ Tennis, pickleball, bowling, or golf equipment
- ☐ Swimsuit and goggles
- ☐ Access to the internet, with endless free exercise resources on YouTube and websites like AARP and the YMCA
- ☐ Exercise/movement/dance videos
- ☐ Memberships to a gym or community center through my workplace, health insurance, Silver Sneakers

Spaces and Places

- ☐ Sidewalks and walking paths
- ☐ Parks and other outdoor areas
- ☐ Community centers, gyms, and fitness centers
- ☐ Park districts and Ys
- ☐ Places of worship
- ☐ Kitchen and bathroom counters
- ☐ Soft carpet or exercise/yoga mats
- ☐ Stairs—even one step
- ☐ Hallways and walkways

MOVE Benefits

Some types of exercise and movement can help you manage health concerns better. Heart-pumping, heavy breathing movement (cardiovascular exercise) and strength, stability, and stretching movements have so many benefits.

Heart-pumping, heavy breathing movement (22 or more minutes a day) helps with:

- Cardiovascular health (that's why it's called cardio)
- Blood pressure management
- Blood cholesterol management
- Prediabetes and diabetes management
- Osteopenia and osteoporosis management
- Stress relief
- Weight management
- Digestion (keeps food moving)
- Arthritis
- Aches and pains
- Better sleep

Strength, stability, and stretching movement (11 or more minutes a day) helps with:

- Osteopenia and osteoporosis
- Arthritis
- Age-related muscle decline (sarcopenia)
- Weight management
- Blood cholesterol management
- Prediabetes and diabetes management
- Better sleep
- Improved range of motion in joints and muscles
- Better posture
- Improved blood circulation
- Injury prevention
- Stress reduction and relaxation
- Better balance and coordination
- Improved digestive health
- Enhanced daily activities of life, such as holding, picking up, and lifting

How Do You Like to MOVE?

Now that you've taken inventory of your MOVE assets, ask yourself a few questions to help direct your movement options into action. Remember, your whys for moving are your own and may be different from the reasons and motivations of others. Psychologist Ralph Trimble poses this question in his book *Motivation for Exercise*: "What positive benefits would you like to receive through a fitness lifestyle?"

- What movement would you like to do more of in your day?
- What new activities would you like to try?
- Where can you do these activities?

- What activities make you feel good when you do them?
- Are there friends, family members, or colleagues who might join you in activities?

You get the idea. Do what you like to do, explore new ways to move your body, and make it fun. We're always more consistent with exercise when we like what we're doing. That's what keeps us moving for a lifetime.

Moving More and Better

As you get more active and discover how exercise best fits into your day (it's up to you), consider boosting the time you spend being active a little more each day. The more active you become, the more you may be able to do—and the more you may want to do, because you're reaping the many benefits of consistent exercise. As you move more or try new activities, you may experience some muscle soreness as your body gets used to changes in your physical activity and adapts to a new routine.

Consider working with an exercise professional like an exercise physiologist or certified personal trainer to hone your movement program.

"An exercise professional can help you identify and define your ideas and goals, help you create effective, safe, and enjoyable activity programs and plans, and give you support and encouragement along the way," says Laura Rooney, PhD, exercise physiologist and clinical associate professor at Marquette University in Milwaukee. She says exercise professionals can also help you find new and interesting ideas for activity and exercise and answer questions you might have about exercise or how to adapt activity to your specific needs.

Look for a certified exercise professional. Start with the US Registry of Exercise Professionals (*usreps.org*). Check with your local Y or fitness center to find certified exercise experts. If you have specific questions about your health and adding exercise to your lifestyle, talk with your physician or health-care provider first.

No Limits to Moving

If you have physical limitations, anxiety about exercising around others, a diagnosed disability, or other challenges to being active, you still have plenty of movement opportunities. If you need mobility assistance from a wheelchair, cane, or walker, or need to modify your movement to accommodate vision or hearing concerns, you can still stay active. Health professionals, including physical therapists or occupational therapists, can help you choose movements that are best for you.

Evidence-based programs that assist individuals with a specific diagnosis can help you start or continue to get your move on. Boxing classes for persons with Parkinson's disease and bone-strengthening exercises to help manage osteoporosis are just two examples. To find additional resources, check the National Center on Health, Physical Activity, and Disability at *nchpad.org*.

MOVE Opportunities

Take a few minutes to think about your current MOVE opportunities. Consider all of the activities you currently enjoy or would like to do, or tasks you'd like to complete during the day:

☐ Walking   ☐ Gardening

☐ Dancing   ☐ Mowing the lawn

☐ Playing with kids or grandkids   ☐ Raking leaves

☐ Washing the car

- ☐ Cleaning the house
- ☐ Swimming
- ☐ Water exercise classes
- ☐ Biking
- ☐ Bowling
- ☐ Running
- ☐ Lifting weights
- ☐ Exercising with resistance bands
- ☐ Using exercise equipment like an elliptical trainer or stationary bike or rower
- ☐ In-person exercise classes
- ☐ Online exercise class
- ☐ Exercise and dance videos
- ☐ Hiking
- ☐ Frisbee and frisbee golf
- ☐ Golfing
- ☐ Playing on playground equipment
- ☐ Playing sports
- ☐ Basketball
- ☐ Volleyball
- ☐ Soccer
- ☐ Hockey
- ☐ Tennis
- ☐ Table tennis
- ☐ Pickleball
- ☐ Badminton
- ☐ Softball
- ☐ Martial arts (karate, taekwondo, tai chi)
- ☐ Boxing and kickboxing
- ☐ Riding horses
- ☐ Yoga
- ☐ Pilates
- ☐ Barre and dance classes
- ☐ Canoeing
- ☐ Kayaking
- ☐ Paddleboarding
- ☐ Sailing
- ☐ Ice skating
- ☐ Downhill and cross-country skiing
- ☐ Snowshoeing
- ☐ Curling
- ☐ Exploring

Just MOVE!

10

Everyday Moving and the One-Week MOVE Plan

Your body works best when you sit less and move more. Let's explore simple ways you can do that throughout the day to boost your health and well-being. In this chapter, you'll learn how to keep moving when you're on the go, out and about, at home, at work, and on the run. Perhaps you use a standing desk, or even do some of your work while on a treadmill. You can work movement into your day in many ways.

You'll find a week of sample MOVE plans with examples for getting in 22 or more minutes of heart-pumping exercise and 11 minutes or more of strength, stability, or stretching each day.

Akin to how you plan what you eat over meals and days, plan how you move the same way. Moving more every day equates to moving more over the whole week. That turns into moving more over months and years of your life. That's the goal.

You can maintain an active lifestyle by choosing activities that work for you, blending movement with nature, being with people you enjoy, and building activities into your day so they become second nature to you. Because there are so many health and well-being benefits to moving with heart-pumping exercise and strength, stability, and stretching, you have a lot of options.

Plan your move opportunities the night before, when you also take your two minutes to consider what you'll eat the next day. Taking that moment to think about the day ahead makes you more apt to stay active and eat well.

Of course, you may have days where your schedule is disrupted, and sometimes your schedule may be unpredictable. You might also have days where your energy level or mood make it hard to be as active as you would want. We all have days like that. Adjust your movement plans to fit your day, and don't worry if sometimes your plans don't work out at all. Keep your options open and look for ways to work in some movement where you can. When you have many ways to MOVE, it's easier to stay active every day.

One-Week MOVE Examples

Your one week of MOVE examples is set up to provide you with a variety of options for moving your body with the 2211 plan. The most important point is to move in ways you enjoy and can be consistent about doing regularly. You may also want to try different MOVE options in the one-week plan to see which you like. The one-week plan is based on the 2211 MOVE principles for moving at least 33 minutes a day on most days:

- Purposefully move your body in ways you enjoy that get your heart beating deeper and faster than usual (aerobic exercise) for at least **22** minutes a day.

- Do strength, stability, and stretching activities for at least **11** minutes a day.

- Move often during the day, getting up at least once an hour to walk, stretch, or take a movement break.

Sample Day 1

- 22 minutes (or more) of heart-pumping movement: 22 minutes (or more) of brisk walking with a friend or family member, or on your own, if you prefer.
- 11 minutes of strength, stability, or stretching: 11 minutes of the "Wait to Bake" strength routine while a meal is cooking (explained soon).
- MOVE breaks during the day: Get up and move around for 5 minutes every hour.

Sample Day 2

- 22 minutes (or more) of heart-pumping movement: 22 minutes (or more) of bicycling outside or on a stationary bicycle. You can do this all at once or break it up into two or three short bursts.
- 11 minutes of strength, stability, or stretching: 11 minutes of tai chi with an online program.
- MOVE breaks during the day: Get up and move around for 5 minutes every hour.

Sample Day 3

On days when you're pressed for time, use your movement breaks from sitting to accumulate 22 minutes of heart-pumping exercise and 11 minutes of strength activities. Here's an example:

- 22 minutes (or more) of heart-pumping movement:

  Break 1: 5 minutes of marching and going up and down stairs.
  Break 2: 5 minutes brisk walking.
  Break 3: 5 minutes of dancing to your favorite music.

Break 4: 5 minutes of brisk walking.
Break 5: 5 minutes of marching and going up and
   down stairs.

- 11 minutes of strength, stability, or stretching: 11 minutes of gentle yoga and stretching before bed.
- MOVE breaks during the day: Get up and move around for 5 minutes every hour.

Sample Day 4

- 22 minutes (or more) of heart-pumping movement:

   11 minutes (or more) of a brisk walk with a friend or
      family member or on your own, if you prefer.
   11 minutes (or more) of a brisk walk around the parking lot, mall, or grocery store before shopping.

- 11 minutes of strength, stability, or stretching: 11 minutes of strength exercises using resistance bands while listening to your favorite music.
- MOVE breaks during the day: Get up and move around for 5 minutes every hour.

Sample Day 5

- 22 minutes (or more) of heart-pumping movement: 22 minutes (or more) of an in-person or online dance class.
- 11 minutes of strength, stability, or stretching: 11 minutes of "Take a Break at Your Desk" routine (explained soon).
- MOVE breaks during the day: Get up and move around for 5 minutes every hour.

Sample Day 6

- 22 minutes (or more) of heart-pumping movement: 22 minutes (or more) of a group exercise class or video or playing pickleball, tennis, or table tennis.
- 11 minutes of strength, stability, or stretching: 11 minutes of yoga or tai chi.
- MOVE breaks during the day: Get up and move around for 5 minutes every hour.

Sample Day 7

Use your sitting breaks to gain cardiovascular and strength benefits throughout the day.

- 22 minutes (or more) of heart-pumping movement:

  Break 1: 5 minutes of brisk walking.
  Break 2: 5 minutes of an online exercise video break.
  Break 3: 5 minutes of brisk walking.
  Break 4: 5 minutes of an online exercise video break.
  Break 5: 5 minutes of brisk walking.

- 11 minutes of strength, stability, or stretching:

  Break 6: 5 to 6 minutes of strengthening with hand weights.
  Break 7: 5 to 6 minutes of wall push-ups, sit-ups, and squats. Aim for 10 wall push-ups, 10 sit-ups, and 10 squats with a 1-minute break. Repeat once.

- MOVE breaks during the day: Get up and move around for 5 minutes every hour.

Strength, Stability, and Stretching Routines

Wait to Bake Strength Plan

You can easily do this 11-minute strength break when you're in the kitchen, waiting for a meal to cook in the oven or on the stove, or even when you have a sheet of cookies baking in the oven.

- 1 minute of marching
- 10 counter push-ups
- 10 counter squats
- 30 seconds balance on the left leg (holding the counter if needed)
- 30 seconds balance on the right leg (holding the counter if needed)
- Repeat 2 more times

Take a Break at Your Desk

This 11-minute program provides a great break from working on the computer or sitting in one position.

- Walk for 2 minutes, stretching out your legs.
- Stand next to a wall and extend your arms as high as you can, stretching up for 30 seconds. Relax and repeat.
- Hold onto a stable chair without rollers, desk, or counter to brace yourself. Swing one leg from front to back slowly, 20 times. Switch legs.
- Continue bracing yourself. Stand on one leg and slowly move the opposite leg in small circles behind you for 20 clockwise circles, and 20 counterclockwise circles. Change legs and repeat.

- Sitting in your chair, place your feet flat on the floor. Roll your shoulders forward for a count of 20. Roll your shoulders back for a count of 20.
- Bracing yourself, get up and down from your chair 10 times, being careful to use your legs to push you up and down.
- Repeat one more time.

Find the videos of these 11-minute breaks and more MOVE ideas at *eatmovegroove.com*.

Ways to MOVE Throughout the Day

One of the best parts of EAT MOVE GROOVE is that you can use the simple 2211 framework to support both eating and moving. The more you use the framework, the easier it is and the more it becomes your norm. Remember that moving throughout the day, no matter where you are or what you are doing, is the key. Keep moving and keep maximizing your well-being.

- Have someplace to go. Check the mail. Walk around your floor at work. Take the long route to the restroom.
- Follow the music. Do you have a favorite artist? Make your movement break fun by moving to music. Music can help us clear our minds, and it can motivate us to dance and move with purpose.
- Take a housework break. Vacuuming may be a chore if you have to do it all at once. But how about taking a vacuum break every few days and vacuuming a room or two? Before you know it, your 5-minute break has whirled by. If you've got some other chore to do, such as emptying the dishwasher or putting in a load

of wash, do it as a movement break. You'll feel good, boost your activity, and make a dent in your chores.

- Look for stairs. By going up and down stairs, you give your body an energy boost as you rev up your engine faster than walking on a flat surface. When I'm working at home, I often go up and down the stairs as part of my 5-minute break. No stairs? Start your walk with 30 seconds of getting up and down out of your chair to boost your heart rate.

- If you're home, plan a short strength, stretching, or stability break in a specific room. You might go to the kitchen to refill your coffee, and while there, engage in a 5-minute kitchen routine. Keep resistance bands and hand weights in the living room and use them for a movement break during the day or in the evening while watching television.

- Play with your pets. Throw a ball and play fetch, play tug, or play hide-and-seek. Take your pet for a short walk. We feel good when giving attention to our pets, and they are always happy to see us.

- Stand up and stretch. If you work at a computer or are in a seated position for a lot of the day, your body needs to open up and stretch out at least once an hour.

- If you have places to go, get off the bus or train one stop early, park farther away from your destination, or walk or bike instead of driving or taking public transportation whenever you can. Those short opportunities to move your body really add up.

- Move while you cheer. Do you have kids, grandkids, or neighbor kids you take to a rehearsal, sports team practice, or game on a consistent basis? Take advantage of opportunities to move while the kids do their thing. Get up from the bleachers between innings of a baseball or softball game, during halftime of a soccer match, or every quarter during a basketball game. If you're in a gym, take a walk around the school during breaks, going up and down stairs. If outside, make a loop around the field during breaks. You're taking care of yourself while supporting your loved ones.

- Keep a pair of sneakers in your car just in case you have an opportunity to move. You might find yourself sitting in the car or outside of school waiting for kids to finish activities. Or you might be waiting to fill a prescription. Take a walk instead of sitting down. Put on your sneakers and go.

- Shop with your personal well-being in mind. At the grocery store or elsewhere, take one or two loops around the outer aisles before beginning your shopping. If you can, aim for 11 minutes of walking before you begin shopping. Use a cart if that helps with balance. You can easily add 10 to 15 minutes of activity to your day.

- Track your steps with an inexpensive pedometer, fitness tracker, or free step tracker phone app. This can be a great motivator. You can quickly see how several 5-minute walking breaks (about 500 steps each at a brisk pace) really add up over the day. You'll tally 2,000 steps or more with 22 minutes of brisk walking in your day.

Link Activity Breaks to Your Daily Routine

Finding well-being cues throughout the day to link to movement can help you be active several times a day. When you begin to associate one activity with another, it becomes easier to remember to do them on a consistent basis. Before you know it, you don't have to think about moving, and you move more as second nature.

- What if every time you brush your teeth, you also do a minute of balance exercises at the bathroom vanity? You're already used to brushing your teeth, so piggyback a minute of balancing on one foot, trading off after 30 seconds. Hold on to the vanity if you need to.

- How about taking a minute to stretch your legs and do toe raises when you wash your hands? After washing, stand on your tiptoes, and then rock back to your heels; repeat 10 times. Brace yourself by holding onto the sink to stay stable.

- Do you have a meeting with a colleague or a phone call to make? How about setting up a "walk and talk" meeting? Or plan for a catch-up call and walk while you enjoy a conversation with friends or family. You're completing a task that needs to be done, but at the same time, you offer yourself a dose of well-being.

- Add a warm-up to your warm-up. For example, when I heat up food in the microwave, I like to stand at the kitchen counter and do deep knee bends or wall push-ups while I wait for the food to warm. It may only be for a minute, but I'm reminded to get moving every time I put food into the microwave and shut the door.

- At night, make a habit of taking 5 minutes to gently stretch your body before getting into bed. Turn the lights down, put on soft music, and take a few deep breaths before you gently stretch. This helps prepare you for a sound night's sleep.

PART III

How to GROOVE

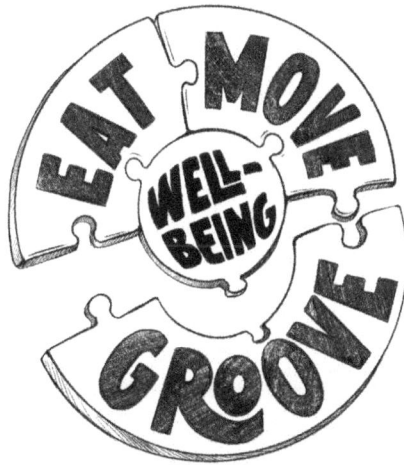

11

How to GROOVE: The 2211 GROOVE Framework

The 2211 simple lifestyle plan is set up with three equally important foundations: what you EAT, how you MOVE, and how you GROOVE. GROOVE is the inner workings of the plan. Finding your GROOVE and staying in the GROOVE keeps your healthy lifestyle going over days, weeks, months, and years.

GROOVE is the positive reinforcement and reflection that helps you take care of yourself and develop the 2211 lifestyle into your lifelong norm. By incorporating all three aspects of the plan each day in simple, practical, doable ways, you'll find the pieces to the puzzle that support your commitment.

Like EAT and MOVE, GROOVE supports your personal well-being. You will utilize the GROOVE techniques to take care of yourself every day. When you're in your GROOVE, you find it easier to EAT and MOVE in ways that work for you. You may have been on and off diet or exercise plans throughout your life. Maybe you've picked up this book because you're looking for a positive approach to taking care of yourself. Or perhaps you're seeking the complete opposite of a restrictive diet plan, the kind that in the past you only stayed on for a short while before it just became too much.

In the earlier parts of this book I helped you understand how to eat better and how to move to enhance your health and well-being. With support and reinforcement, eating and moving well each day can become your norm. As you do this, you're getting in your groove—you're taking care of yourself each day, and, in turn, extending the length of your life and your healthy years.

In the next chapter you'll explore 22 ways to get your GROOVE on and find simple, daily options for supporting yourself.

When we asked people what they currently do (and what they need support doing) with the GROOVE part of their well-being, many areas stood out as important. At least 50 percent of respondents from our 2211 survey noted these key action areas as being especially beneficial:

- Participate in activities that bring me JOY
- Do activities that RELIEVE STRESS
- Spend time with people who make me HAPPY
- Spend time OUTSIDE
- TURN TO FRIENDS OR FAMILY when I need to talk or need help
- TAKE TIME TO RELAX and recharge
- Do acts I find MEANINGFUL, PURPOSEFUL, and IMPORTANT
- Get enough SLEEP
- Stay on top of HEALTH CHECK-UPS

- Challenge my BRAIN
- Practice GRATITUDE
- RESET myself when life gets in the way of my well-being

How can you get into your personal groove? How can you make simple changes in your life that let you do the things you want and need to do on a consistent basis? Here's an example with some of the benefits you may receive.

You might have a very busy work life during the week. But on the weekends, you get some time for yourself. You intentionally set up a catch-up walk at a local park every weekend with a dear friend. You look forward to it during the week, and you receive a myriad of benefits from this weekly event.

First, you get to spend time with someone you enjoy. Second, you can de-stress by going through your week and talking about anything that's on your mind. Third, you're enjoying nature and the world around you. Fourth, you're moving your body in a way that feels good to you. Fifth, this serves as a positive way to reset for the coming week. You're a super groover.

You can put into place dozens of simple practices in your life to help you GROOVE every day. These daily supports help you build EAT MOVE GROOVE into your daily life.

Start by giving yourself positive reinforcement.

You've picked up this book. That's a great start. You're learning about a new, simple approach to taking care of yourself in a positive way. Give yourself a hand.

Every step you take that moves you toward well-being, no matter how small, is a step forward. Stop and give yourself positive reinforcement each time you do something that enhances your health and well-being.

Let's look at other ways to get your GROOVE on.

GROOVE at the Grocery Store

Think of grocery shopping not as a chore but as an opportunity to groove by being thankful. When I put fruits and vegetables into my cart, I look at the cart and thank myself. It may sound a bit odd to you, but honestly, I'm grateful to be able to have a cart with all kinds and colors of produce in it. I realize it's a privilege to be able to purchase produce.

That moment of reflection, of positivity, is meaningful and reinforces the other positive choices I make for the well-being of myself and my family. Adopting the simple 2211 lifestyle is a cause for celebration. You're taking positive action to enhance your health and well-being.

In his book *Atomic Habits*, author James Clear says, "The more pride you have in a particular aspect of your identity, the more motivated you will be to maintain the habits associated with it."

I couldn't agree more. See yourself as a 2211 lifestyle groover. Envision yourself as someone who is utilizing this book and this program to enhance your personal well-being. Own it. Then, it's easier to do it.

Subscribe to EAT MOVE GROOVE

Be a 2211 subscriber on the *eatmovegroove.com* website. This unlocks the key to becoming a member of the EAT MOVE GROOVE community. You'll find all kinds of ways to support your well-being lifestyle with tips, recipes, articles, movement ideas, relaxation exercises, and fun ways to eat, move, and groove through life.

"Your habits shape your identity, and your identity shapes your habits," according to Clear. Making a commitment to your health and well-being also makes you a health and well-being believer. Making a commitment to the **2211** lifestyle plan makes you a **2211** community member. Kudos to you.

Give Yourself 2211 Well-Being Reminders

When we give ourselves **2211** well-being reminders through-out the day, we're much more likely to act on them and adopt the changes we want to make in life. Reminders don't have to take a lot of time or energy—they just have to be consistent.

Reminders are an essential part of finding our groove. When we live with intention, supporting our efforts to take care of ourselves and giving ourselves permission to find ways to boost our health and well-being, we're getting in our groove.

Here are a few examples of ways I support my personal EAT MOVE GROOVE lifestyle each day by living with intention.

2211 Fruit Bowl Fueling

In our kitchen, we keep a big fruit bowl on the kitchen counter. Not only is the bowl a pleasant, colorful piece of kitchen art to look at, it's also one of our **2211** well-being reminders to include 2 cups of produce with meals.

Each morning, when we make breakfast, the fruit bowl makes it so easy to grab an orange or banana and add it to the meal. At lunch, I often slice an apple or pear because it's right there within reach.

At night, when we're cleaning up the kitchen, the fruit bowl is in sight, reminding me to refill it for the next day. By doing so, I don't have to think about whether I've got fruit ready for the next day. It's right there within reach.

2211 Daily Protein Boost

Here's another example of a simple 2211 well-being reminder I put into place over a decade ago to help me eat more protein at breakfast.

At the time, in my mid-forties, I was doing a lot of learning, writing, and speaking about the importance of building and maintaining muscle strength as we age. I began looking more closely at what could be done to stay strong and lessen age-related muscle loss. This happens to all of us as we get older, but by strengthening our muscles and eating well, we can minimize the losses. Part of what I learned helped fuel this book.

Several research studies at the time investigated how protein was consumed during the day. Typically, in American diets, we tend to eat meals with the lowest amount of protein at breakfast, and the highest amount of protein at the evening meal. Why is this a concern? When we skimp on protein at breakfast, we miss getting enough protein to keep our muscles strong by refueling them after sleeping. This is a critical time to eat more protein, not less. Protein helps to turn on muscle growth during the day, especially after an overnight fast. The bottom line: Find ways to get more protein at breakfast to start your day.

A recent study backs up this idea. Researchers reviewed three-day food records of nearly 500 adults fifty-five years of age and older. The average protein intake at breakfast was 13 grams for women and 15 grams for men. For lunch, the average intake of protein was 18 grams for women and 20 grams for men. But for dinner, the average intake was 34 grams for women and 38 grams for men. Only 1 percent of the participants met the protein intake goal for breakfast.

Increasing protein intake at breakfast by just 10 grams (about 1.5 ounces of protein) helped participants meet total protein intake throughout the day. That's the equivalent of one and a half eggs, about 2 Tablespoons peanut butter, or about half a cup of Greek yogurt. This is one simple strategy for potentially enhancing strength and decreasing muscle loss and frailty as we age.

So how did this play out for me years ago? Let's go back to the year 2010. With this knowledge, and a self-assessment of my own typical breakfast intake, I realized I was falling short on protein at breakfast. I decided to use a simple nutrition piggyback for my breakfast. I thought about a food or drink I consumed every morning and looked for a way to enhance it. The answer: coffee.

I changed my coffee routine so that I drank my coffee with more milk. All I had to do was add a half cup of warm milk to my morning mug to get an extra 4 grams of protein. I drank two mugs each morning, so I was adding 8 grams of protein every morning while enjoying my coffee.

It's that simple. It was an easy change that became my daily routine. Since that time, I've changed the milk to a high-protein version, which boosts the protein even more.

You could modify this protein piggyback in many ways, depending on your preferences. You might try soy milk, pea milk, or cashew milk, which are three plant-based milk options that can boost morning protein intake.

Here are more simple, inexpensive ways to add protein to breakfast:

- Spread peanut butter, almond butter, or any nut butter on toast.
- Keep hard-boiled eggs in the fridge and add one to your breakfast.
- Add a scoop of yogurt to your fruit salad.
- Warm up a piece of leftover pizza.
- Choose a high-protein cereal.

- Add a slice of cheese or a scoop of cottage cheese to your breakfast.
- Choose a high-protein wrap for your breakfast burrito.

Starting our days with intention also has other positive implications besides helping us stay strong with more protein in the morning. Any time we opt into a well-being opportunity early in the day, we feel good about it all day. That's an important lasting benefit for implementing wellness opportunities in the morning if your schedule allows.

2211 Morning Walk Team

We have two playful dogs at home. They're so much fun and have so much energy. We're all happier when the dogs get a good walk in the morning. I get the benefit of being outside and taking in nature, which nurtures my soul, and get to spend time with my dogs, which starts me off on a positive note.

The bonus from this nature and movement piggyback is I get in my morning 22-minute (or more) walk. It's a super win-win that gives me a sense of accomplishment early in the day.

Positivity Break

When I'm writing at my desk, I take regular breaks to reenergize myself, get up and move, and refocus. One of the ways I do this is to take a positivity break.

I keep a sign near my desk that says "Be Bold! Trust Yourself." It's a reminder to me that I can get the work done, try new things, be creative, and keep my goals in sight. When I take a break and say the words aloud several times, it provides me with a positive reminder to believe in myself as I author this book and move into new territory with EAT MOVE GROOVE.

Write yourself a positive note as a reminder to believe in yourself and carry on. What uplifting or inspiring message do you most need to hear? Put it where you'll see it a few times a day. Take the time to pause and read your affirmation aloud. It works.

Well-Being Reminders

What does your day look like? Are there times during the day when you can piggyback an EAT, MOVE, or GROOVE habit? Where can you build in your personal 2211 well-being reminders? When we have a behavior reminder or cue, we're much more likely to follow through with the behavior on a consistent basis.

Some simple reminders that can help you implement the 2211 plan into your daily life include these:

- Complete your 2211 2-minute miracle plan each night before bed.
- Start your day with three deep breaths.
- Keep a full fruit bowl in plain sight on your kitchen counter.
- Cut up fresh vegetables and keep them in the refrigerator in a see-through container.
- Wash your salad greens in advance or buy prewashed salad mixes.
- Prepackage 2211 lunches for the next day right after dinner.
- Make a grocery list every week using the 2211 grocery list.
- Shop for groceries every week to ensure you have plenty of produce and other healthy food available.

- Cook in bulk on the weekends.
- Set out your sneakers at night so you're ready to take a morning walk.
- Pack your fitness bag every night if you exercise outside of home.
- Charge your step tracker at night so you're ready to go in the morning.
- When working, set an alarm to remind you to get up and stretch.
- Take a walk or move your body in a way that feels good to you before or after a meal.
- Schedule a catch-up and move walk with a friend each week.
- Take time to connect with nature every day.
- Post positive reminders of your worth around the house.
- Listen to your favorite music.
- Be still and be grateful for each day.

Now that you've gotten the idea about how GROOVE supports your EAT and MOVE plan on a daily basis, let's dig more deeply into 22 ways you can get your GROOVE on.

12

22 Ways to Get Your GROOVE On

As research expands beyond the EAT and the MOVE pieces of personal well-being, we learn just how many different aspects of life contribute to overall health and wellness. For this chapter I've chosen 22 aspects of life that make a positive impact on our well-being. Some of these are based on our 2211 survey. Others are founded in decades of science.

1. Make a plan

Create your own 2-minute miracle you can rely on to support your well-being every day. Take a few minutes to set yourself up for a great tomorrow. This can mean doing a few small things each night, so you are prepared to eat and move in ways that support your well-being the next day. What does this look like for your personal lifestyle, situation, and daily routine? Your 2-minute miracle could include any of these ideas:

- Set out my walking shoes.
- Choose clothes that feel good on me.
- Fill the fruit bowl on my table.
- Clear my desk.
- Prepare a space for a meditation break.
- Pack a 2211 lunch.
- Fill my water bottle.
- Place my exercise bands in plain sight.
- Cut up fresh veggies.
- Plan out my 2211 produce and proteins for the next day.

Think about the fast, small things you can do before you go to bed to make it easier for you to EAT, MOVE, and GROOVE tomorrow. This is a gift you can give yourself every night to support your personal well-being.

2. Link your day to 2211 activities

Imagine small ways you can develop links in your day to 2211 activities. Think of it as setting up no-brainers around your 2211 lifestyle plan. Here are some ideas to try:

- While you brush your teeth, practice standing on one foot at a time, holding onto the counter if you need to. This adds a few minutes of balance exercises to your day. You can also do this in the kitchen whenever you have a few moments, such as waiting for the microwave to heat something up.

- When you sit down for a meal, take three deep breaths. Inhale through your nose, and exhale through your mouth. You relax and get prepared for your meal.
- Park in the last row of the parking lot. That way, you get in some extra steps just by walking to and from your destination.
- Keep a squeeze ball handy in your workplace and in the kitchen. When you get a chance at work or sit down to eat, do twenty squeezes with each hand. This keeps your fingers and hands strong and flexible and helps relieve stress.
- Do 10 sits and stands (they take about a minute) before you sit down for a meal. Make sure you have a sturdy chair and a table or counter to hold onto, if needed. Sit down and get up slowly and deliberately. Doing this three times a day can boost your leg strength considerably. Plus, you'll be well on your way to 11 minutes of strength, stretching, and stability.

3. Find your "community of generosity" and give back

Whether you help neighbors, volunteer with a community program, or lend a listening ear to a friend, taking time to help others can make a powerful, positive impact in your life. Seek ways to reach out to others. Finding a good fit for you can be a real game-changer when it comes to your personal well-being.

Volunteering in a meaningful way on a consistent basis can:

- Provide a sense of purpose to your life
- Offer the chance to learn a new skill
- Connect you with others in your community
- Boost your mood and attitude

- Reduce stress by releasing "feel good" hormones
- Nurture a sense of overall well-being

When I moved to Milwaukee years ago, I kept hearing about a unique food pantry that was doing amazing things. For decades previously, I had volunteered at food pantries and food banks. Ever since I was a child and witnessed my mother's commitment to standing with people in need, this has been important to me. Everyone deserves to eat enough good, wholesome food.

When I first volunteered at Kinship Community Food Center in Milwaukee, I immediately felt the community spirit I had heard so much about. Their motto is "Everyone has something to give, and everyone has something to receive." In other words, I go to Kinship to volunteer, but I receive just as much as I give.

Kinship Executive Director Vincent Noth notes that this "community of generosity" fosters meaningful opportunities to both give *and* receive. Being involved in this program has positively impacted my well-being and the well-being of many of my students in significant ways.

Being a part of something bigger than yourself that is truly changing lives for the better brings meaning to life.

Are there volunteer opportunities in your community where you can be of help to others while gaining the benefits of finding your community of generosity? Untapped volunteer opportunities may be waiting for you.

4. Laugh often

Tickling your funny bone may do a lot more than simply offer a moment of humor in your day. In fact, researchers are finding that laughter has a positive effect on your well-being. Whether it's reading something funny, watching funny videos online, enjoying your favorite comedy show on television, or being silly with friends and family, laughter is definitely great medicine.

Laughter can improve your psychological well-being, boost your mood, decrease depression, lower anxiety, and reduce stress. The physical action of laughing can induce chemical changes in your body that not only reduce stress but may increase pain tolerance and improve your immunity.

Some practitioners think laughter is so beneficial to your health that it should be prescribed to patients. A laughter prescription might even specify the frequency, intensity, time, and type, just as an exercise prescription does. This makes so much sense. Studies show that laughter can help lower blood pressure and help manage blood sugar levels. Studies also find that people who laugh more are also likely to be healthier overall.

One simple way to ensure you have laughter as a part of your life is to plan laughter breaks in your day. Here are some examples:

- Watch your favorite comedy show on television.
- Catch a short comedy video on the internet.
- Tell a joke to a friend.
- Read something funny.
- Talk with a friend or family member who always makes you laugh.
- Listen to a funny podcast while you're commuting or preparing dinner.
- Play with kids. There's always something to laugh about.

5. Practice positivity

Many research studies have documented the benefits of having a positive outlook, where you see the good things in your life rather than the negatives. Having a positive outlook helps you enjoy life to the fullest, and it also impacts your overall health.

In one study of people with a history of heart disease, those with a positive outlook were one-third less likely to have a heart attack or be hospitalized than those with a more negative outlook. The positive outlook was noted by assessing several factors, including the participants' optimism, energy level, and cheerfulness. Having a negative outlook can weaken the immune system and increase inflammation in the body, which could contribute to heart disease.

We feel better overall when we're positive than when we're negative. Practicing positive thinking can lead to better coping skills in times of stress or when events get extra challenging in our lives. We can manage situations better when we keep a positive mindset and a clear head.

Even if you're already a positive person, you can enhance your positivity:

- Accept that change is a part of life and is bound to occur over and over. Resisting change can take a toll on you.

- Make it a point to be around positive people. If you're around others who are positive, you're likely to feel more positive about the world around you.

- Reframe your thinking. When you're in a difficult or stressful situation, reframe it so you see the positive. When you're dealing with something hard, for example, instead of focusing on what could go wrong, focus on what new opportunities it presents. This takes some practice.

- Practice positive self-talk. Sometimes we say negative things to ourselves that we wouldn't dream of saying to others. Move to positive self-talk by being accepting, nonjudgmental, encouraging, gentle, and caring to yourself, just as you want to be with others—and hope they will be to you.

6. Be with your people

Research from the Blue Zones—those areas of the world where people tend to live longer, healthier lives—links longevity to having a healthy social network. Especially when we have hardships in our lives, being in community with people we trust provides the emotional support needed to make it through challenging situations. Inevitably, we will have struggles and difficulties, and moving through these in community is a boost to our well-being.

Staying socially engaged supports your brain health just as much as exercise and healthy eating do. It's strongly recommended by the Global Council on Brain Health, a collaborative group of researchers and other experts convened by AARP. Social engagement also provides comfort, meaning, and a feeling of inclusion and community.

"If you're feeling isolated or are in a new environment, one way to find your people and build a community is to participate in service that supports issues and causes you care about. You may be serving alongside them and collaborating to support the health and well-being of others and the community as a whole," says Ben Trager, PhD, community building expert at the University of Wisconsin–Milwaukee.

One important way to stay engaged is to keep in touch with people important to us. You don't have to travel to connect with them. Sending a note or card in the mail, texting, emailing, calling, and video chats are all ways to stay connected.

In your own neighborhood, you can connect with friends to stroll in a nearby park, take a walk, attend a local event, or just have coffee together. The key concept here is the joy of friendship.

7. Practice mindfulness

With its roots in Buddhist meditation, mindfulness is defined as a calm mental state achieved by focusing your awareness on the present moment. Mindfulness invites you to acknowledge and accept your feelings and thoughts without judgment. I think of mindfulness as a way to be respectful of ourselves and listen to ourselves. To me, it means taking a step back to pause and honor what my mind, heart, spirit, and body are telling me.

Practicing mindfulness can lead to better management of anxiety and depression. Research shows that in some cases it may be as helpful as taking medication. In one study of 276 adults with untreated anxiety disorders, for example, incorporating an eight-week mindfulness-based stress reduction program worked as well as a commonly prescribed anti-anxiety medication.

Practicing mindfulness can be helpful for improving clarity and focus, managing stress, easing pain, promoting better sleep, boosting the immune system, and managing blood pressure and diabetes.

Mindfulness techniques are easy to learn. You can easily use them in your day to be more aware and mindful, anywhere and anytime. To start, try these practices:

- **Body scan mindfulness:** Find a quiet, peaceful place. Lie on the floor or get into a comfortable position in your chair. Relax your body. Starting with your head, focus on each part of your body, moving down the body. What do you notice? How does each part of your body feel? Be aware of any feelings or sensations that come forward as you give each part of your body some time and attention.

- **Awareness break:** Find a comfortable position in which to sit, lie down, or relax. Close your eyes. What do you hear? What feelings do you notice in reaction to the sounds you hear? Take a deep breath and take in the sounds. Release your breath and release any tension you're feeling along with the breath.

- **Explore free guided meditations:** You can find a wide variety of free guided meditations and classes online and in apps such as Calm, Insight Timer, Healthy Minds Program, and Smiling Mind. Some are as short as one minute, while others take you through a series of meditative exercises. These options provide supportive, gentle instruction and a way to let go for a few minutes each day. You'll find links to guided meditations at *eatmovegroove.com*.

8. Be grateful

The effect of having a grateful outlook on our psychological and physical well-being has been studied for years. The research shows that a conscious focus on our blessings in life can have emotional and interpersonal benefits. When we can take the space and time to be grateful, even for the smallest things in life, it positively impacts us.

People who practice gratitude in their daily lives tend to be more optimistic, have a higher sense of purpose, and feel more positive about the world around them. Practicing gratitude can lead to better relaxation and sleep. Those in a grateful mindset often feel less stressed and more able to manage tasks at hand.

"It doesn't have to be anything big. It's about seeing things through the lens of what's going well in our lives," says Mindy Meiering, MSW, an expert on the benefits of practicing gratitude. As Meiering notes, there's always something to be grateful for. It might be as simple as a good night's sleep, or that the air you breathe feels crisp and fresh when you breathe it in on your way to work in the morning. "Inclining our minds toward what *is* working and what *is* going well is the secret to embracing gratitude. If you build that gratitude muscle when things are going well, this helps you to build emotional resilience that can be supportive when challenges arise," says Meiering.

How can you practice gratitude daily?

Keep a gratitude journal. This can be as simple as writing down one thing you are grateful for in the day. The process of thinking about and writing down something you feel good about in your day is a great start. Taking a moment to note what we're grateful for can help us feel better about our lives, even prompting us to be more active, practice better self-care, and stay more optimistic about the world.

Focusing on your blessings in life plays a key role in enhancing personal well-being. Begin by focusing on one person in your day who has done something positive for you or for someone else. Be mindful of that effort.

Another simple way to boost gratitude on a daily basis is to use the five-finger method. Count five things you are grateful for on one hand. This is a calming practice to put into your schedule when you hit the pillow before falling asleep. Take a few deep breaths, be grateful, and relax.

9. Love the animals

During the COVID-19 pandemic, there was something missing at the home of Norma and Dick Graves in Houston. They had always been a dog family, raising their three kids with dogs and enjoying the company of pets. For the previous ten years, however, they hadn't had a dog because they spent a lot of time traveling once they retired and had more time to be on the road.

Their daughter Julie, who is a physician, thought they were too isolated during the pandemic. Julie heard about a puppy who was overlooked and the runt of a litter. Before long, Pepper, a Miniature Schnauzer, joined the family, much to the elation of the Graves family.

Dick walks Pepper three to four times a day. In the evenings, Pepper jumps up to snuggle in the chair with Dick when they settle in to watch television and relax.

"We missed having a dog more than we knew. It's hard to duplicate that unconditional love anywhere else," notes Norma.

In our household, we agree. Every time we walk into our home, we are covered with love from our two dogs, Boo and Mango. It doesn't matter the time of day, whether we're in a rush or have all the time in the world, or what kind of mood we're in. They are there, ready to greet us and show their love and devotion to the simple fact that we exist. We have a lot to learn from our pets in this regard.

Spending time with animals is so nourishing, whether it's petting our furry friends, taking them (and us) on a walk, or just snuggling close with our pets to watch our favorite shows. Animals help us create routines in our lives and can be a motivator to get us up to move frequently during the day. When they need to go out, it's usually also time for us to get up and stretch, move our bodies, or get a dose of fresh air. What's good for them is good for us.

We might enjoy playing with our pets and laugh at the funny things they do, but there is more to this story. Being around animals and caring for pets is good medicine, maybe better than medicine. Coexisting with animals has been linked to a myriad of benefits, including:

- Decreased blood pressure
- Decreased levels of stress hormones
- Enhanced mood

- Decreased loneliness
- Reduced anxiety and depression
- Increased feelings of support
- Enhanced mobility by boosting physical activity

Even if you don't own a pet, you can still harness the positive power of animals. When you take a walk, listen for singing birds, the chatter of squirrels, or enjoy the pets you see walking nearby with their owners. Volunteer at an animal shelter or sanctuary to make a positive difference in the lives of animals—and support your own well-being at the same time.

10. Sleep well

Getting enough high-quality sleep (seven to nine hours a night) is central to maintaining a healthy mind and body. Sleep helps manage stress and anxiety, helps balance hormones, restores tissues and muscles, and keeps our minds sharp. Sleep affects many aspects of brain functioning, such as creativity, learning, memory, decision-making, focus, and concentration.

One way to think about sleep is that it's your preparation for the day ahead. Just as you plan for a healthy breakfast by keeping the right foods on hand, plan for a good night's rest to help you start out on the right foot in the morning.

The key to a good night's sleep is appropriate sleep hygiene:

- Keep your bedroom cool. You'll sleep better if you don't get too hot during the night. Use a fan or air conditioner if needed. Choose loose-fitting, lightweight sleepwear.

- Finish your last meal two hours before you go to sleep. This gives your body time to move food along, so you don't feel too full when bedtime comes. This also helps prevent nighttime heartburn and reflux.

- Keep fluids to a minimum after 8:00 p.m. to reduce nighttime trips to the bathroom.
- It may take up to ten hours for caffeine to get completely out of your system. To keep caffeine from coffee, tea, or other sources from preventing sleep, lay off caffeine for up to ten hours before your usual bedtime to help you get a good night's sleep.
- Make time to unwind before bed. Turn your electronics off at least an hour before bedtime. This frees up time to read, listen to calming music, spend quality moments with loved ones, or journal.
- Stay active. Being active during the day helps your body get ready for rest at night.
- Start your day with sunlight. Seeing natural light early in the day, even if it's just for a few minutes to get some fresh air and morning rays, helps keep your body clock in sync. That way, your body also knows when it's time to sleep.

Sleep is a pillar in our health. Whether you want to live longer and healthier or just feel more energized and excited to take on the day, research shows that optimizing sleep is the way.

11. Practice self-compassion

Practicing self-compassion is one of the most important tools we have. We all need to take care of ourselves. Self-compassion helps us build stronger relationships with ourselves, as well as with others, and has been linked to lower levels of anxiety and depression. When we practice self-compassion, we also build resilience and build up the foundation of our emotional stability.

What is self-compassion? It's turning compassion inward, according to self-compassion expert Kristin Neff, PhD, the author of *Self-Compassion: The Proven Power of Being Kind to Yourself*. It's about offering care and kindness to ourselves, just as we would to others in difficult times. You might ask yourself what a good friend would say to you when you're struggling.

We all have times when we miss the mark or come up short. The key to practicing self-compassion is to be kind and caring to ourselves even during those times. If we want to change things about ourselves, can we do that in a way that doesn't cause us harm or negative feelings? We can ask affirming questions like "What got in my way today?" or "How could I do that differently next time?"

As humans, we make mistakes and learn as we go through life. When we offer that leeway to others, we're reminded to do the same for ourselves. We might call that "meeting ourselves with grace and kindness" instead of beating ourselves up over past mistakes.

As we make habit changes, practicing self-compassion is especially important. We all need some trial and error to figure out what works best. That doesn't mean we're doing anything wrong. Instead, now is a time for exploration and growth. Being gentle and kind with ourselves during these times is essential for our health and well-being.

Practice self-compassion daily by opting into these activities:

- When you feel stressed or tired, lie down, close your eyes, and take a few deep breaths to give yourself a self-compassion break. Remember you're doing the best you can every day.

- Write a thank-you note to yourself. Sit down, choose a beautiful card or a lovely piece of stationery. Gently write yourself a thank-you for managing all life has placed in your path. Note a particular time you made it through something especially difficult. Add a note of gratitude for making it through and carrying on. Sign the note with "All my love." Keep it in plain sight as a reminder to thank yourself often.

- Remind yourself that everyone experiences challenges, setbacks, and difficulties as part of the human experience. Our imperfections make us who we are. Embrace your uniqueness in this world.

12. Breathe deeply

What do we do that fosters our health and well-being without even thinking about it? We breathe. Breathing is involuntary, but when we pay attention to our breath, it becomes a magnificent, free tool to find your groove. We breathe an average of 20,000 times a day, so you have plenty of opportunity.

Every time we take a breath, we bring oxygen into our lungs, nurturing our bodies. When we exhale, we breathe out carbon dioxide, letting go of something we can release. This miracle of the human body keeps us alive. It can also help us care for ourselves. When we're aware of our breath, conscious of each time we bring air in and send it out on its way, we draw ourselves into the present moment. Being one with our breath helps us to center ourselves, reminding us that we're alive and here in this present moment.

The simple practice of taking a deep breath can do wonders. When we deliberately breathe in and out in a slow, steady, and mindful way, our nervous system listens. Simply by breathing mindfully, you can lower your blood pressure, decrease your heart rate, and better regulate your emotions. This helps us manage those times when we feel anxious, angry, upset, and out of control. It doesn't mean we won't feel these emotions. It's just that we can handle them better when they come.

To bring more awareness to your breath, try these practices:

- **Three deep breaths:** Whenever you want to refocus, bring yourself back with three deep breaths. Sit comfortably, close your eyes, and notice your feet flat on the floor. In this way, you anchor yourself. Then take three deep breaths, breathing in through your nose and exhaling through your mouth each time.

- **Open breath:** Sit comfortably. Move your shoulders back to open up your chest as full as possible. Put your hands on your belly. Take a deep breath with your mouth open and hold it for five seconds. Exhale through your nose. This is a helpful breath break when working at a desk.

- **Mindful breathing:** Find a quiet place free from distractions. Sit comfortably or lie on the floor. Close your eyes. Think of a word that makes you happy. It might be *joy*, *peace*, or *love*, or any word that resonates with you (sometimes we call this a mantra). Focus on that one word. For one minute, breathe in that word every time you inhale. Envision your body being filled with joy, or peace, or love.

Our breathing is a gift we own. It is a rhythmic reminder of our existence on this earth. It is our personal groove and available to us every minute of every day.

13. Sing, play music, whistle, hum, and snap

No matter if you strum it, play it, feel it, listen to it, or use your own voice to make music, music has a chorus of benefits for your well-being. Listening to and playing music can boost memory, enhance attention, and even improve cognition. That doesn't even account for the sheer joy when we experience music. Music is the universal connector, the universal language we can all understand.

Music can lift our spirits, boost our mood, and move us into a healthier state of mind. It can relax us, rejuvenate us, energize us, and sustain us. Listening to an old tune from happy times can evoke nostalgia and help us heal. Music accompanies our greatest times and our saddest times, and is always there for us, no matter our tastes or preferences.

Beyond its positive impact on emotions and feelings, music offers a myriad of health benefits. It can lower blood pressure and heart rate, boosting overall cardiovascular health, and can help us manage pain, calm us in periods of discomfort, and help soothe our mind and spirit.

According to a 2020 AARP survey of over 3,000 adults aged eighteen and over, those who engaged in music were more likely to self-report their overall health, brain health, and cognitive function as excellent or very good. Listening to music, whether having music on in the background or attending concerts, was linked to a small, positive effect on mental well-being, depression, and anxiety.

You might find music especially enjoyable by trying new ways to experience it:

- **Listen in the dark.** By listening to music in the dark, you tune out the sense of sight. This can allow you to focus more closely on the music and gain greater appreciation.

- **Take a music break.** When you get up every hour to move around, treating your body to a MOVE break, pop on headphones, or turn up the radio, and enjoy a few of your favorite tunes at the same time. You might even want to dance your break time away.

- **Try a new music genre.** We can get caught in our old music ways, listening to the same songs or same type of music from day to day. Branch out into a new genre you're not as familiar with. You might find these new sounds intrigue you—and your brain will thank you. You're learning something new.

- **Take part in a drum circle.** Drumming is simply fun, and it's also good for your brain. Drumming can help relieve stress and boost the immune system, according to the Yamaha Music and Wellness Institute. Joining a drumming circle is also a proven way to build community and foster belonging.

Music can help you get in the groove, focus, soothe sorrows, connect you to others, and provide joy in your life. It's one of the greatest secrets to lifelong well-being.

14. Dig in the dirt

Gardening does wonders for our mind, our body, and our spirit. When you dig in the dirt, you take yourself away from your work, worries, and demands of the day to refocus your mind and your spirit on the tasks at hand in the garden.

Gardening nurtures you in many ways. You're breathing fresh air. You're basking in the warmth of the sun and harvesting vitamin D from the sun's rays. You're also using your nurturing skills to make something grow. The simple act of watering offers an opportunity to focus on your plants and what they need, bringing positive feelings to you.

One of the best things about plants is that you can check on them daily and note the progress. One day, a flower may be completely closed, and the next day, a burst of color meets your gaze. Plants abound with wonder and bring us delight and surprise at every turn.

Gardening can meet your needs whether you prefer time by yourself with your plants or enjoy being social. You can garden in community plots, join gardening clubs, or set up gardening catch-up dates with friends. You choose what you need, and what works best for you, depending on what makes you happy.

Besides the emotional and social benefits of gardening, gardening is real exercise. Gardening may also be linked to boosts in cognitive health.

Here are some easy ways to start digging in the dirt, even indoors:

- **Designate an inside garden in your home.** Take a corner of a room with plenty of light, or set up inexpensive grow lights, and begin with two or three plants that are easy to grow. Try starting with snake plants, spider plants, philodendrons, or corn plants. You'll brighten up your room right away.

- **Grow your own herbs.** Add fresh flavor to your dishes while enjoying watching them grow. Try basil, rosemary, mint, chives, cilantro, and parsley.

- **Set up an outdoor vegetable garden.** Choose a sunny patch in the yard or use containers on a patio or porch. Start with easy-to-grow lettuce, spinach, radishes, kale, and tomatoes.

- **Volunteer to dig in the dirt.** If you don't have space to garden at home, consider volunteering at a local food pantry or food bank garden. You'll be getting all of the benefits from digging in the dirt while fostering food security in your community.

15. Enjoy nature

Nature is vast in beauty and the well-being benefits it provides. Being in tune with nature is an important way to care for ourselves. It might mean feeling gentle rain on your face, smelling a fragrant flower, walking through a city park, or paddling across a serene lake in the woods. Research backs this up. In one study that followed 20,000 people, those who spent an average of twenty minutes a day in nature gained a boost to their health and well-being.

"That's why we feel so much better after getting a dose of vitamin N, or vitamin Nature," says Abby Check, health and wellness coach in Asheville, North Carolina. She says spending time outdoors is one of the most available avenues for enhancing your health and well-being. Whether you open your window and let the fresh air inside, take a break to walk around the block, or enjoy a hike in the woods with friends, nature nurtures.

Here are some of the ways Mother Nature can take care of you and help you get your groove on in the great outdoors:

- Being in nature can improve your mental health. By focusing on the beauty at hand, it helps to clear your mind, enhance your concentration, and foster a sense of well-being. Embracing nature is associated with reduced anxiety and depression.

- Enjoying time in nature can boost the immune system by increasing the activity of our immune-enhancing cells.

- When we take a break from our daily routines and get outside, we can boost our creativity and come back to our work or demands of daily life with a refreshed approach. Fresh air can lead to fresh ideas.

- Being in nature may even lower blood pressure. In Japan, the practice of forest bathing (*shinrin-yoku*) or immersing yourself in the calming atmosphere of forests and other natural areas, has been associated with reducing blood pressure and lowering stress.

- Breathing fresh air out in nature and exposing our bodies to the wonders of natural light can help us rest better at night. Time spent outside, especially when we are moving, can help regulate our circadian rhythms, resulting in better sleep.

16. Embrace spirituality

Spirituality can mean different things to different people. To some, it is based on finding a sense of connection to something greater than yourself. It may be founded on a personal, individual exploration of the depths of your spirit, finding balance and harmony, even transcendence. To others, it may mean participating in a spiritual community or organization. Or perhaps spirituality is a sense you receive when in tune with the natural world.

No matter your personal belief system, having a spiritual practice can be one way to find your groove.

Studies have linked the positive effect of spirituality on physical health, mental well-being, quality of life, and utilizing coping skills to manage life. A 2022 research review of the link between spirituality, health, and managing illness found that for healthy people, spiritual community participation, notably religious service attendance, was associated with healthier lives, less depression, and greater longevity. Whether in community with others, or on your own, embracing your spiritual side can provide well-being benefits. The key is to find what feels authentic and is meaningful to you.

- Create a sacred space in your home. Find a corner in a room or a quiet place where you can rest, reflect, and rejuvenate.

- Combine meditation or focused breathing with tuning in to your spiritual self.

- Connect with yourself by taking a few minutes out of your day to consider your spiritual well-being. Add a moment of gratitude and then return to your task at hand.

- Be patient with yourself and offer yourself grace as you explore your spiritual side.

17. Listen to your body

Listening to your body and being aware of your body's signals is an important way to feel your groove. Sometimes life gets going so fast that we don't slow down enough to do this. But our bodies know what we need, and when we take the time to listen, we can consistently practice self-care.

With the EAT MOVE GROOVE plan, listening to your body is paramount. You do this by eating foods that taste good to you, moving in ways that feel good to you, and supporting your personal well-being in ways that resonate with you. By listening to your individualized needs and preferences, you are supporting your well-being every day.

One way to listen to your body is to identify the signals your body is sending you. For example, if you're extra tired one day, perhaps you need rest instead of working late. If you're feeling overwhelmed, it may be time to step away, take some deep breaths, and refocus. Being physically hungry for a meal may feel different from wanting to eat out of boredom or because you feel stressed. Being in touch with your emotions as well as the physical feedback your body provides will help you stay on your well-being path.

Laura Becker, RDN, owner of Louga Fitness & Nutrition in the Denver area, encourages listening to your body's cues to learn to feel and understand different sensations. She says, "Listening to your body and practicing intuitive eating has been linked to more positive body image, more positive eating practices, and less depression in women."

By thinking of the EAT MOVE GROOVE plan as a flexible foundation for your health instead of a rigid diet or exercise program, you're listening to what your body needs. Some days you may feel hungrier and need to eat more; other days, you may not. Some days you may be more active; other days, you may need more rest. Maintain the feeling of flexibility with yourself, nurturing your needs each day.

18. Play like a kid—just for fun

When was the last time you played just for the fun of it? I hope it was today. Embracing play has many wonderful side effects. When we were children, we would gain all the benefits of running, jumping, stretching, laughing, being with friends, exploring nature, and soaking in the sun all in one by playing outdoors. There's no reason to stop playing just because we're adults.

In fact, climbing a tree, wading through a creek looking for frogs, sailing homemade paper boats across a pond, or zooming in and out of play equipment with kids are all incredibly good for us. Even the simple task of figuring out where the best hiding spots are in a game of hide-and-seek tweaks our minds and our bodies. We must think differently, consider how to solve problems, improvise, and be creative. All these experiences stimulate the brain, boosting cognitive well-being.

When we engage in play, we boost our mood and release "feel good" hormones that help manage anxiety and depression. We also release endorphins, which are chemicals in the brain that help us feel less stressed. When we play, we release the neurotransmitter dopamine, which boosts our feeling of well-being and happiness.

Playing with others, whether it's table tennis or cards, has social benefits. Playing with others fosters our connections and provides opportunities to build positive experiences and fun memories to think back on. In work situations, adding play has been found to boost job satisfaction and enhance innovation. Playing is good for us, no matter where we play or how old we are. Here's how to play more:

- Take a play break from work. Give yourself a five-minute break to put on your favorite music and dance by yourself—or with anyone who will join in the fun.

- Think back to yourself as a kid. Which board games did you enjoy the most? Bring back your favorites and invite your family and friends together for a game night and make it a regular event.

- Explore your artistic side with painting, pottery, crafting, drawing, or creative writing. Sign up for acting classes or join a community theater group. Mixing play with being creative helps us relax and feel good about what we are creating.

- Play in ways that also boost your physical well-being. How about jumping on a trampoline, playing on a pogo stick, walking on stilts, hula hooping, or jumping rope?

19. Let it go

As humans, we have the power to do so much good in the world. But we can also hurt others or cause them pain, sometimes without even realizing it. When we've been hurt by the words or actions of another, it can be challenging to let go of that pain, especially if our experiences were traumatic and caused long-lasting damage. Letting go and forgiving others doesn't mean we excuse the harm done to us, or necessarily forget it. But such actions allow us to move on with our lives, and in this way, we support our well-being.

Each of us has our own path to roll through when it comes to finding forgiveness for the pains in our past. Wherever you are on that road to healing, understanding the power of forgiveness can help you step back and see how holding onto this pain holds you back as you move to embrace personal well-being.

Forgiving and letting go might mean something a little different to each of us, depending on our experiences. Forgiving is the act of making a purposeful, intentional decision to let go of hurt and pain. I visualize forgiving as unzipping the main pocket of a heavy backpack and unloading the hurt and pain I've been carrying. Then I think about how light the backpack is now, and how I don't have to carry that weight any longer. For me, this way to see the release of the pain is helpful when I strive to move on from a negative experience.

Letting go of the pain, bitterness, anger, and grudges we hold against others can open us up to receive the many benefits of practicing forgiveness, including:

- Improved self-worth
- Improved clarity in our lives
- Less hostility toward others
- Improved mental health
- Enhanced empathy
- Healthier relationships
- Improved immune system
- Lowered blood pressure
- Improved heart health
- Enhanced emotional healing

Is there something that has been eating at you that you'd like to move past? That's the right place to start. Looking inward to find what's bothering you and making an intentional effort to let it go can free you and open up a place for healing and enhanced well-being.

20. Learn and grow

No matter where you are on life's journey, there's always room to learn new skills, explore new ideas, and gain expertise in new areas. And grow. When we commit to learning new things, we tell our brain to rev up and get ready for incoming information. Learning and engaging in new activities keeps the brain sharp, boosting cognitive health.

When we learn new things, gain new experiences, and push our boundaries to get outside of what's comfortable for us, we expand our personal capabilities. This leads to enhanced self-worth and self-esteem—in other words, we feel good about what we've accomplished. We also expand our perspectives, gain new insight from others, and enhance our empathy for the life experiences of others when we learn and grow.

Learning new things also allows us to function at a higher level in our ever-changing world. Gaining an understanding of innovative technologies, new developments, and ever-present societal shifts helps us stay engaged and involved. By cultivating a lifelong curiosity about the world, we also enhance personal feelings of well-being and self-understanding.

Challenge yourself to learn and grow so you can find your groove every day. Here's how:

- **Read and listen.** Find books, magazines, blogs, articles, podcasts, shows, programs, and lectures that interest you.
- **Acquire a new skill.** Maybe you've always wanted to learn more about basic car maintenance, plumbing, or

planting and harvesting food from your own garden. Now is the time.

- **Transfer your skills to make a difference.** Take a skill you've already mastered and use it to teach others or help those in need.

- **Be curious about others.** Ask questions and try to understand where others are coming from and how their life experiences have shaped them.

21. Reach out

Taking care of your well-being includes reaching out to friends, family, and professionals when you need guidance and support, when life feels too overwhelming, when you feel stuck, or when you're dealing with situations that are difficult to manage on your own. Reaching out to others shows strength, as you're willing to ask for help when you need it.

Seeking support from others helps you know you're not alone and can ease the stresses you may be experiencing in life. Sometimes we may feel as if we're the only ones going through specific challenges, but there are others we can learn from, gain support from, and move forward with.

Building and maintaining a strong support system you can rely on through life is an important well-being foundation. Having a robust support system supports you in these ways:

- Better coping skills
- Feelings of connectedness to others
- Reduced depression
- Less anxiety
- An ability to move through challenges
- A longer, healthier life

One way to build a strong support system is to take inventory of the people in your life now. Who can you reach out to? How can you expand that circle with family, friends, community groups, support groups, health and well-being coaches, mental health professionals, or online support?

22. Stay connected to the 2211 online community

I hope you will also join the 2211 online community. I invite you to log on to *eatmovegroove.com* and check out all the ways you can gain support for your well-being lifestyle. Learn about new ways to EAT, MOVE, and GROOVE. Go beyond this book and get EAT tips and recipes, MOVE tips and opportunities, and find lots of ways to GROOVE every day. Sign up for the EAT MOVE GROOVE email newsletter for more ideas delivered directly to your inbox.

I look forward to seeing you there.

References and Resources

Chapter 3

Eat-Lancet Commission Summary Report (2019). https://eatforum.org/eat-lancet-commission/eat-lancet-commission-summary-report/.

Feeding America. https://www.feedingamerica.org.

Leenders, M., Sluijs, I., and Ros, M., et al. (August 15, 2013). Fruit and Vegetable Consumption and Mortality: European Prospective Investigation into Cancer and Nutrition. *American Journal of Epidemiology*, 178(4): 590–602, https://doi.org/10.1093/aje/kwt006.

National Center for Complementary and Integrative Health. https://www.nccih.nih.gov/.

Oldways Whole Grains Council. https://www.wholegrainscouncil.org.

Oyebode, O., Gordon-Dseagu V., Walker A., et al. (2014). Fruit and Vegetable Consumption and All-Cause, Cancer and CVD Mortality: Analysis of Health Survey for England Data. *Journal of Epidemiology & Community Health*, 68: 856–862. https://jech.bmj.com/content/68/9/856.

Produce for Better Health. https://www.fruitsandveggies.org.

Reynolds, A., Mann, J., Cummings, J. et al. (February 2, 2019). Carbohydrate Quality and Human Health: A Series of Systematic Reviews and Meta-Analyses. *The Lancet*, 393(10170): 434–445, https://www.thelancet.com/journals/lancet/article/PIIS0140-6736(18)31809-9/fulltext.

Rock, C. L., Thomson, C., Gansler, T., et al. (2020). American Cancer Society Guideline for Diet and Physical Activity for Cancer Prevention.

CA: A Cancer Journal for Clinicians, 70: 245–271. https://doi.org/ 10.3322/caac.21591.

US Department of Agriculture and US Department of Health and Human Services. Dietary Guidelines for Americans, 2020–2025. 9th edition. (December 2020). https://www.DietaryGuidelines.gov.

Wang, D., Li, Y., and Bhupathiraju, S., et al. (April 2021). Fruit and Vegetable Intake and Mortality: Results from 2 Prospective Cohort Studies of US Men and Women and a Meta-Analysis of 26 Cohort Studies. *Circulation,* 143(17): 1642–1654. https://doi.org/10.1161/ CIRCULATIONAHA.120.048996.

Wang, F., Baden, M.Y., and Guasch-Ferré, M. et al. (April 8, 2022). Plasma Metabolite Profiles Related to Plant-based Diets and Risk of Type 2 Diabetes. *Diabetologia,* 65: 1119–1132. https://doi.org/10.1007/ s00125-022-05692-8.

Chapter 4

Academy of Nutrition and Dietetics. https://www.eatright.org/.

The American Heart Association Diet and Lifestyle Recommendations. https://cpr.heart.org/en/healthy-living/healthy-eating/eat-smart/ nutrition-basics/aha-diet-and-lifestyle-recommendations.

Evert, A., Dennison, M., and Gardner, C. et al. (2019). Nutrition Therapy for Adults with Diabetes or Prediabetes: A Consensus Report. *Diabetes Care,* 42(5): 731–754. https://doi.org/10.2337/dci19-0014.

Chapter 9

American College of Sports Medicine Physical Activity Guidelines. https://www.acsm.org/education-resources/trending-topics-resources/ physical-activity-guidelines.

American Heart Association Recommendations for Physical Activity in Adults and Kids. https://www.heart.org/en/healthy-living/fitness/ fitness-basics/aha-recs-for-physical-activity-in-adults.

Colberg, S., Sigal, R., and Yardley, J. et al. (November 1, 2016). Physical Activity/Exercise and Diabetes: A Position Statement of the American Diabetes Association. *Diabetes Care,* 39(11): 2065–2079. https://doi. org/10.2337/dc16-1728.

Currier B., Mcleod J., and Banfield L., et al. (2023). Resistance Training Prescription for Muscle Strength and Hypertrophy in Healthy Adults: A Systematic Review and Bayesian Network Meta-Analysis. *British Journal of Sports Medicine*, 57(18): 1211–1220. https://bjsm.bmj.com/content/57/18/1211.

Diaz K., Howard V., and Hutto B., et al. (October 3, 2017). Patterns of Sedentary Behavior and Mortality in US Middle-Aged and Older Adults: A National Cohort Study. *Annals of Internal Medicine*, 167(7): 465–475. https://pubmed.ncbi.nlm.nih.gov/28892811/.

Lee, D. H., Rezende, L. F. M., Joh, H-K. et al. (July 25, 2022). Long-Term Leisure-Time Physical Activity Intensity and All-Cause and Cause-Specific Mortality: A Prospective Cohort of US Adults. *Circulation*, 146(7): 523–534. https://www.ahajournals.org/doi/10.1161/CIRCULATIONAHA.121.058162.

National Center on Health, Physical Activity and Disability. https://nchpad.org.

National Public Radio "Body Electric" podcast. https://www.npr.org/series/1199526213/body-electric.

Saint-Maurice P. F., Graubard B. I., Troiano R. P., et al. (2022). Estimated Number of Deaths Prevented Through Increased Physical Activity Among US Adults. *JAMA Internal Medicine*, 182(3): 349–352. doi:10.1001/jamainternmed.2021.7755.

US Department of Health and Human Services, Physical Activity Guidelines for Americans, 2nd edition. https://health.gov/sites/default/files/2019-09/Physical_Activity_Guidelines_2nd_edition.pdf

US Registry of Exercise Professionals. https://usreps.org/.

Chapter 11

Clear, J. (2018). *Atomic Habits: Tiny Changes, Remarkable Results: An Easy and Proven Way to Build Good Habits and Break Bad Ones.* New York: Avery.

Verreijen, A. M., van den Helder, J., Streppel, M. T., et al. (April 2021). A Higher Protein Intake at Breakfast and Lunch Is Associated with a Higher Total Daily Protein Intake in Older Adults: A Post-Hoc Cross-Sectional Analysis of Four Randomised Controlled Trials. *Journal of Human Nutrition and Dietetics*, 34(2): 384–394. doi:10.1111/jhn.12838.

Chapter 12

Balboni, T. A., VanderWeele, T. J., and Doan-Soares S. D., et al. (2022). Spirituality in Serious Illness and Health. *JAMA*, 328(2): 184–197. doi:10.1001/jama.2022.11086.

Blue Zones. http://bluezones.com.

Global Council on Brain Health. https://www.aarp.org/health/brain-health/global-council-on-brain-health/.

Global Council on Brain Health. (2020). Music on our Minds: The Rich Potential of Music to Promote Brain Health and Mental Well-Being. https://www.aarp.org/content/dam/aarp/health/brain_health/2020/06/gcbh-music-report-english.doi.10.26419-2Fpia.00103.001.pdf.

Hoge, E. A., Bui, E., and Mete, M., et al. (2023). Mindfulness-Based Stress Reduction vs Escitalopram for the Treatment of Adults with Anxiety Disorders: A Randomized Clinical Trial. *JAMA Psychiatry*, 80(1): 13–21. doi:10.1001/jamapsychiatry.2022.3679.

Hunter, M. R., Gillespie, B. W., and Chen, SY-P. (2019). Urban Nature Experiences Reduce Stress in the Context of Daily Life Based on Salivary Biomarkers. *Frontiers in Psychology*, 10: 722. doi:10.3389/fpsyg.2019.00722.

Li, S., Hagan, K., Grodstein, F., and VanderWeele, T. (March 2018). Social Integration and Healthy Aging Among US Women. *Preventive Medicine Reports*, 9: 144–148. doi.org/10.1016/j.pmedr.2018.01.013.

Louie, D., Brook, K., and Frates, E. (June 23, 2016). The Laughter Prescription: A Tool for Lifestyle Medicine. *American Journal of Lifestyle Medicine*, 10(4): 262–267. doi: 10.1177/1559827614550279.

Self-Compassion with Dr. Kristin Neff. https://self-compassion.org/.

Acknowledgments

To my wife, Audrey, you encouraged me to write this book, build the EAT MOVE GROOVE program, and follow my dream. Thank you for your unyielding support and belief in me. Special thanks to our kids Georgia, Isa, and Lindsay, for lending a listening ear, providing feedback, and offering creative suggestions for the book and to my big, wonderful, extended family, especially to Janet, who provides steadfast support and encouragement.

I am fortunate to have collaborated with such incredible colleagues on this project. I am especially grateful to Lisa Burgoon, whom I have worked with for over thirty years, for your dedication to reading every word in this book and collaborating in such a positive, consistent way. I appreciate Laura Rooney, Carol Kennedy-Armbruster, Ann Swartz, Karen Miyoshi, Stacey Krawczyk, Jan Seeley, Melinda Flegel, Dee Ann Valles, Mindy Meiering, Heather Fink, Peggy Gates-Wieneke, Kelly Reynolds, Abby Check, Patti Miller, Tatiana March, Doris Montgomery, Hannah Antonson, Leah Seidel, and Ben Trager for your detailed review, feedback, and expertise.

Special thanks to the incredible professionals in the nonfiction book writing and marketing arena I have gained so much from, especially Beth Godbee, Stephanie Chandler, Carla

King, Tracee Garner, Mary Catherine Jones, Stacy Ennis, Steve Friedman, Dale L. Roberts, and Joanne McCall. Special thanks to marketing and small business experts Scott Clanin, Jess Johnston, Daniel Lanza, Laura Gmeinder, Heather Wentler, and Madeleine Wolske. Thank you to my developmental editor Sheila Buff, copy editor and book coach Sandra Wendel, designers Kirsten Dennison and Marko Markovic, illustrator Irina Burtseva, and proofreaders Mary Fleming and Kristen Roberts. Your guidance, expertise, and collaboration have been invaluable.

Thank you to the first 2211 focus group who tried out the early EAT MOVE GROOVE program, provided valuable reflections, and helped ignite the movement back in 2019. I am especially grateful to Kelly Tetting, Wendy Huddleston, Robyn Deterding, Tracy Oles, Lora Vega, and Courtney Chramowicz. Thank you to my amazing Waldorf Warriors focus group for your ideas, honesty, and energy: Tracy Keninger, Stephanie Price, Carletta Nymeyer, Tammy Naig, and Kim Sheda. I also appreciate the thousands of individual clients, group participants, corporate workshop attendees, and online participants who helped build, simmer, and nurture EAT MOVE GROOVE.

This book wouldn't be possible without the reviews and feedback from friends, early readers, and cold readers, especially Julie Larson, Erna and Larry Todd, Karyn Miller, Peg Penwell, Sarri Danker, Sheila Wenger, Kristy Skoglund, Susan Buntin, Caron Barnhardt, Cindy Butkovich, Pete Fernandes, Paula Smith, Jean and Bob De Vita, Terry Gantert, Sue Margheim, Dennis Cockrum, Joel Brotherton, and Norma Graves. Thank you!

Thank you to my amazing EAT MOVE GROOVE interns who have helped with research, evaluated recipes, created social media, and assisted with the book launch. I especially appreciate the contributions of Laura Becker, Iris Grems, Gracien Jules,

Isabel Breitbach, Jalynn Brown, Kendra Dantoin, Leah Hoefert, Maddie Saltiel, Madison Bauer, Saige Kearns, Summer Hausz, Lilia Tregoning, Brooke Overholt, Catt Clarke, Dani Davis, Elly Flaherty, Erin Pawelczyk, Veronica Buis, Kayla Lammy, Bella Buettner, and Autumn Young. I am also grateful for the help of former students Reese Slobodianuk, Doug Bartel, Elizabeth Lindquist, Rachel Hahn, Jenny Pethan, Morgan Jenswold, Pafoua Xiong, and Alexis Krenke. Students make the best teachers.

To the reader: Thank you so much for reading this book. I am truly grateful. I hope *EAT MOVE GROOVE* and the online resources are a support for you on your wellness journey. It was a life-long dream to research and write this book for you! Please consider sharing *EAT MOVE GROOVE* with friends, family, and colleagues and writing a review online. Your feedback and support are always appreciated and allow me to continue to do what I love to do—spread simple, positive, doable ways to boost health and well-being.

About the Author

Susan (Susie) Kundrat, MS, is a Registered Dietitian Nutritionist and wellness expert and the founder of the lifestyle program EAT MOVE GROOVE.

An enthusiastic and award-winning instructor, Susie is a clinical professor emeritus in the Joseph J. Zilber College of Public Health at the University of Wisconsin–Milwaukee and an adjunct lecturer with the University of Illinois Urbana–Champaign Food Science and Human Nutrition Department and Walla Walla Community College.

Susie was the consultant sports dietitian with the Milwaukee Bucks and US Speedskating. Susie worked in many roles at the University of Illinois Urbana–Champaign. She was the sports dietitian for the Fighting Illini athletic teams, manager of the SportWell Center, and outreach dietitian with the Functional Foods for Health program.

She served as consultant sports dietitian with Northwestern University, Bradley University, and the University of Evansville athletic programs. She and Michelle Rockwell, PhD, RD, developed RK Team Nutrition to train nutrition experts around the country on optimal sports nutrition education programming for athletes of all ages.

For ten years, Susie ran Nutrition on the Move, Inc., a nutrition and wellness consulting business located in Strawberry Fields Natural Food Store in Urbana, Illinois. She served as media dietitian, was the nutrition expert on the WILL 580-AM monthly call-in show, and worked with clients, organizations, and groups to boost wellness with current science-based nutrition and health recommendations.

Susie earned an associate degree from Waldorf University, where she was a three-sport first-team all-region athlete in basketball, softball, and volleyball and was inducted into the Waldorf University Athletic Hall of Fame. She earned her BS in dietetics from Minnesota State University–Mankato, where she was named Honor Athlete. She completed a dietetic internship at Boston's Beth Israel Deaconess Medical Center and a master's degree in human nutrition from Iowa State University.

Susie is the recipient of the Sports, Cardiovascular, and Wellness Nutrition (SCAN) Award for Excellence, the Collegiate and Professional Sports Dietitians (CPSDA) Service Award, and the UW-Milwaukee College of Health Sciences CARES Award, Leadership Award, and Byoung Kim Teaching Excellence Award. She was honored with the Illinois Young Dietitian of the Year Award through the Illinois Academy of Nutrition and Dietetics.

As a consultant with a zeal for well-being, Susie has worked with consumers and athletes of all ages to optimize health, well-being, and sports performance with simple, practical, doable nutrition and wellness solutions. She collaborates with corporations, organizations, and institutions to maximize health and well-being and help clients thrive with her trademarked EAT MOVE GROOVE program.

For more information on Susie and EAT MOVE GROOVE, or to book a keynote presentation with Susie, scan the QR code or go to *eatmovegroove.com.*

What experts say about *EAT MOVE GROOVE*

"If you think food is meant to be enjoyed, appreciated, and explored, this book is for you.

"If you think exercise is meant to be fun, joyful, and achievable, this book is for you.

"If you want a lifestyle that makes you feel good about how you are living, this book is for you.

"Congratulations to Susan Kundrat for writing an upbeat, positive, and science-based guide for everyday people who want to have more energy, feel better, and maintain good health for the long run."

Nancy Clark, MS, RD, CSSD,
author of *Nancy Clark's Sports Nutrition Guidebook*
and owner of Sports Nutrition Services, LLC

"The last book you'll ever have to buy to guide your healthy lifestyle. Susie teaches us how to eat simply and joyfully, how to move in positive ways, and how to nurture our inner selves. This trifecta is a winning recipe for health and wellness."

Jan Colarusso Seeley, Director,
Christie Clinic Illinois Race Weekend

"*EAT MOVE GROOVE* is your GPS for helping you prioritize, personalize, and realize your chews, moves, and grooves so you can strive and thrive with a focus on your 'can do' for you."

Leslie Bonci, MPH, RD, CSSD, LDN,
owner of Active Eating Advice by Leslie Bonci Inc.
and co-founder of Performance365

"I had the opportunity to work with Susie many years ago at the University of Illinois. She is an outstanding prac-ademic as she can apply research to practice directly with the use of simple methods that help you live your best life. I highly recommend *EAT MOVE GROOVE* to anyone who seeks contemporary evidence-based nutrition and well-being solutions. It is the best simple science book on eating, moving and grooving for life I have read. You will LOVE it!"

Carol Kennedy-Armbruster, PhD,
co-author, *Fitness and Well-Being for Life*

"*EAT MOVE GROOVE* is a refreshing guide full of important information to help us eat better, move more, and become healthier. Susie does a great job of taking the science and blending it with years of experience to create a plan for adopting a healthier lifestyle."

Ann Swartz, PhD,
co-director of the Physical Activity and Health Research Lab
at the University of Wisconsin-Milwaukee

"What makes this book so unique is how Susie integrates simple, scientifically-based concepts in nutrition, fitness and wellness with a positive and practical approach to daily eating, exercise and living well. The three-part daily well-being solution is easy to adapt to your lifestyle to foster your well-being goals and fuel your personal success plan for life."

Lisa Burgoon, MS, RD,
former Director of the Minor in Leadership at
the University of Illinois Urbana-Champaign

"Anyone looking for a practical, daily way to meet their health and wellness goals—whether to have more energy, feel better, manage their weight, enhance productivity at work, or boost stamina on the pickleball court—will find the EAT MOVE GROOVE foundation is a flexible and positive way to do it."

Heather Fink, MS, RD, LD, CSSD, CLT,
author, *Practical Applications in Sports Nutrition,* 7th edition,
founder of Nutrition & Wellness Solutions

"Susie has a way of capturing and communicating accessible and achievable ways for living well. Her EAT MOVE GROOVE philosophy is spot on! Using the simple and easy to remember **2211** formula takes the guesswork out of what we can do to make better choices every day."

Stacey Krawczyk, MS, RD,
Food Systems and Wellness Marketing Expert

"If you're looking for sound, science-based health and wellness advice to put into practice today and every day, *EAT MOVE GROOVE* is the book for you. Susan takes the science and makes it applicable in an energetic way, whether speaking to groups of 500, training health professionals, or maximizing well-being and productivity in corporate settings."

Michelle Rockwell, PhD, RD, Senior Research Associate and
Assistant Professor, Department of Human Nutrition, Foods,
and Exercise, Virginia Tech Carilion School of Medicine

"*EAT MOVE GROOVE* reframes eating and moving in a positive, uplifting way. We can eat and move again as acts of nourishment and love! The **2211** framework is science made simple, and it's easy to follow without becoming a burden."

Laura Rooney, PhD, Clinical Associate Professor, Exercise Science, Marquette University and owner of Laura Rooney, LLC, Coaching and Consulting

"Bringing GROOVE into the mix highlights community and relationship building as key components of a holistic plan for well-being. This refreshing take on wellness is one that considers our deep need for connectedness and familiarity in a comprehensive yet totally accessible way."

Ben Trager, PhD, Interim Director of Community Engagement and Experiential Learning, University of Wisconsin–Milwaukee

"This book is a beautiful testament to the fact that there is no one-size-fits-all program for living our healthiest lives. Solidly incorporating the latest science and research, Susie gives us a simple, flexible approach for eating healthfully, incorporating regular movement into our lives, and cultivating mental and emotional well-being in a variety of ways that support our overall well-being. A practical roadmap that is easy-to-follow and will support anyone who wishes to nurture their health and wellness!"

Mindy Meiering, LCSW, Licensed Therapist, Professional Life Coach and Certified Mindfulness Teacher, author/creator of the Rainbow Bridge Pet Loss Deck

"EAT MOVE GROOVE is a positive, practical, inclusive lifestyle plan, not a diet. You won't go on and off the 2211 plan. It's your invitation to wellness for life because it's science-based and simple to put into practice every day, for everyone."

Connie Diekman, MEd, RD, LD, FADA, FAND,
Food and Nutrition Consultant,
former president of the Academy of Nutrition and Dietetics

"The EAT MOVE GROOVE program can make a positive impact on individuals as well as on companies looking to optimize the health and well-being of their employees. Susan and I have worked together to develop well-being programs for Fortune 500 companies to decrease disease risk, boost fitness and health, and enhance worksite productivity. She is an engaging speaker and an experienced clinician who blends real-world experience with science to make it come alive."

James Di Naso, MS, CSCS, NSCA-CPT
Performance Director/co-owner, Practical Kinesiology Company

"With *EAT MOVE GROOVE*, Susie Kundrat puts the simple back in health. Most of us think we need to move mountains and eat in a very specific way when what we really need are small, simple nudges to get us going; *EAT MOVE GROOVE* does just that!"

Stuart Phillips, PhD, Professor and
Canada Research Chair, McMaster University